I0449015

Fat Trap

Be the size you want once and for all

J.E. Orias

Copyright © 2015 J. E. Orias

All rights reserved, including the right to reproduce this book, or portions thereof in any form. No part of any text or images may be reproduced, transmitted, downloaded, decompiled, reverse engineered, or stored, in any form or introduced into any information storage and retrieval system, in any form or by any means, whether electronic or mechanical without the express written permission of the author.

Disclaimer

The contents of this book are intended to provide helpful information on the subjects discussed. This book is not meant to be used, nor should it be used, to diagnose or treat any medical condition. Please consult with your doctor before embarking on an exercise or dietary programme. The author is not responsible for any specific health or allergy needs that may require medical supervision and is not liable for any damages or negative consequences from any treatment, action, application or preparation, to any person reading or following the information in this book. References are provided for informational purposes only and do not constitute endorsement of any websites or other sources. Readers should be aware that the websites listed in this book may change.

Although the author has made every effort to ensure that information in this book is correct at time of print, the author does not assume and hereby disclaims any liability to any party for any loss, damage, or disruption caused by errors or omissions, whether such errors or omissions result from negligence, accident, or any other cause.

Illustrations by RENÉ BINDSLEV
Contact information:
E-mail: rene.bindslev@jubii.dk
Website: www.rb-tegnestue.com/shop

ISBN: 978-1-326-42685-9

This book is dedicated to my mum and dad.

Notes from the author

Please read chapters in chronological order.
This book does not delve into weight gain due to medical conditions or genetics.

The use of word "diet"

The word "diet" is used interchangeably throughout this book either as a general term for the food we eat, or a special course which restricts a person's eating to lose weight.

Registered nutritionist and qualified fitness instructor J.E. Orias is passionate about sharing her knowledge, research findings and personal experiences to help provide practical and sustainable options to improve health and overall wellbeing.

Contents

Acknowledgement

Thank you to all those I pestered relentlessly for feedback!

Chapter 1

Introduction

Despite being active in my teens, I spent more years than I'd like to remember in the "chubby category" – carrying excess pounds around my midriff. Unable to shake off the extra weight I firmly settled into my "chunky status". I could not get my head around how some of my friends would literally stuff their faces with food, but managed to stay super slim while I struggled just to maintain a healthy weight despite exercising my guts out. Never one to buy into the whole, "some people are just destined to be fat" school of thought, I made it my personal quest to try and truly understand what causes weight gain and how best to keep it at bay – forever!

There's still a misconception that most people who are overweight simply suffer from a large dose of sloth and gluttony – eat too much, move too little.

You can exercise your butt off in the gym, know the calorie content of every morsel of food that passes your lips, have an impressive grasp of calorie burn by activity but still sport a big belly. The thing is, your body doesn't need to retain that many calories to accumulate excess fat and become overweight but, in the same vein, a few knowing dietary and lifestyle changes can promote consistent fat burn and tip the scales in your favour.

When it comes to weight loss many roads can lead to the same place, but who wants to take the scenic route? Having an understanding of the real reasons people gain weight can equip you with the practical know-how to beat the battle of the bulge once and for all while still having a life.

Chapter 2

Keeping topped up

What is it with work colleagues? The mere mention of my desire to upgrade myself to a fitter, leaner, healthier me sends them on a not so covert mission to derail my efforts – to the point of leaving treats on my desk!

If your work environment is anything like mine, between birthday treats, holiday treats and, more recently, Friday treats, temptation to indulge in sugary and salty snacks is all too often round the corner. I even recall a colleague pleading with the usual culprits to stop buying treats or put them on the other side of the office.

We all know what it's like. As soon as you take the first bite the floodgates fly open and before you know it you're debating whether to endure the walk of shame to the "treat zone" for a third visit.

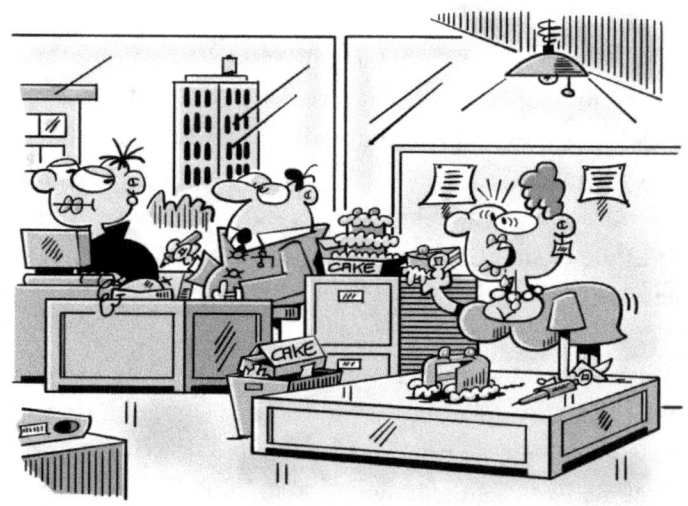

At the risk of sounding facetious, it dawned on me one day that, just because I'm surrounded by cakes, doesn't mean I have to eat them…

When I have my wits about me and I'm stocked up with healthy snacks, every cake and doughnut going no longer seems to be calling my name.

Over time, as we introduce healthier food choices, sugar cravings will subside. The process of getting to this point can be challenging, especially at the beginning, and we truly must want the change more than we want our food vices. Don't get me wrong, the thought of devouring a moist Victoria sponge cake with vanilla ice cream on the side still fills me with a warm fuzzy feeling of anticipation, but I have more control over my cravings now than ever before, and when I do choose to indulge I tend to eat a lot less of it as the anticipation of having a treat usually seems far better than the actual experience.

You are more likely to eat "bad" unhealthy food when you are hungry, as the desire to over indulge in food when hungry is much stronger and harder to control. So one of the key steps to staying strong in the face of temptation is to keep hunger pangs at bay:

1. **Eat quality protein with each meal**. Protein requires more energy and takes longer to digest than carbohydrates (carbs) – helping you feel fuller for longer. Also, our body burns about 20% of calories from protein just to digest it (around 8% of calories form carbs and 2% from fat are burned during digestion)[1]. Glutamine, an amino acid – the building blocks of protein – [not to be mistaken for man-made additive Monosodium Glutamate (MSG)] is a natural appetite suppressant and will help curb cravings. Meat, fish, poultry and eggs contain the highest levels of glutamine. Beans, peas, lentils, milk, yoghurt, ricotta and cottage cheese are also rich sources, while red cabbage, kale and spinach are considered to be some of the more dense vegetable sources of glutamine (see page 80 for suggested protein intake).

2. **Eat 5–6 times a day at regular intervals**. Three meals with 2–3 snacks in-between to ward off hunger. Leaving long gaps between meals can result in low blood sugar levels and encourage cravings which can lead to overeating. Food cravings can often be a sign of nutrient deficiencies, so ensuring that meals are nutritious can give you the strength to pass on a multitude of guilty food pleasures.

In terms of people attempting to sabotage your efforts, I have learned that you don't need to tell all and sundry about your pending quest for a slimmer, healthier you. However, having a like-minded friend or co-worker who is either on a similar journey or simply supportive of your efforts can make all the difference. If no one knows of your mission it can be easy to slip back into old habits. Putting your intentions out there brings an element of accountability. No one wants to be caught chomping on a cream cake minutes after pledging themselves to a life of becoming clean and lean.

<u>Fat trap fact 1</u>
Glutamine is a natural appetite suppressant and can help curb cravings. To keep hunger pangs at bay eat 5–6 times a day – 3 meals with 2–3 snacks in-between and consume quality protein with each meal.

Chapter 3

All calories are not equal

While grabbing lunch out some time ago, I overheard two ladies talking about weight loss. "I'm really chuffed with my eating yesterday. I had breakfast before I left home – around 250 calories – then I was so busy I didn't stop all day, so I grabbed three shortbread biscuits and some orange juice on the train. I think I only had 700 calories for the whole day! I'm really determined this time."

To which the second lady chipped in approvingly, "That's really impressive; so your weight loss plan is going well then?" As I stood there eavesdropping – forgive me ladies, it was for the greater good – two thoughts came to mind: 1. Like many of us, this was not her first attempt at losing weight and 2. Shortbread biscuits and orange juice – really?

I like shortbread biscuits as much as the next person, and everyone already knows that eating too many sugary and processed foods will not do our waistline any favours but, when it comes to the calories we eat, it goes deeper than that. Once food enters our body, **all calories are not equal**, a 500 calorie meal can either be satiating – keeping hunger pangs at bay and assist with weight loss – or leave you ravenous within hours and encourage weight gain. Without this being at the forefront of our mind, the concept of a calorie-controlled diet is questionable.

Chinese people eat more calories than Americans but are slimmer.
A study carried out by T. Colin Campbell, PhD of Cornell University, US in 1990 compared stats of 6,000 adults in China to different countries and, in particular, America. Included in the study were records of calorie intake and body weight. It revealed, when compared to Americans, people from China consumed about 30% more calories yet their body weight was 20% lower[2].

You might be thinking the difference in weight may be due to Chinese people being more active, however, the figures quoted related to the least active group of Chinese (sedentary office workers) compared to the average American who undertakes moderate exercise several times a week[3].

Some may argue that differences in genetics may be the reason for the disparity. However, more recent studies in China have shown a sharp rise in child obesity which experts attribute to a radical change in diet (in addition to reduced physical activity). Historically, despite consuming a high percentage of calories from "carbohydrate foods" such as rice, intake of sugar and total amount of carbs in China have been low with proportion of omega-3 (from fish and fish oils) high. This is a stark contrast to a typical western diet.

Perhaps a closer look at how our body uses food can help provide some additional insight.

Human cells: At a microscopic level, our body is composed of trillions of cells – muscles, bones, skin, hair follicles – all formed from various types of living cells. Every function that our body has and can perform happens at a cellular level. Food we eat is broken down, digested and used by our cells. To function efficiently, cells need to be provided with a variety of nutrients, all of which can play a crucial role in assisting weight loss.

Macronutrients include carbohydrates (sugar compounds), proteins and fats.

Micronutrients include vitamins and minerals.

There are 2 types of vitamins:
Fat soluble vitamins include A, D, E and K. If the body receives more of these vitamins than required, it can be stored in the liver and body fat to be used later. To enable absorption, an adequate amount of fat is required in your diet. Generally, these vitamins will not be lost when food that contain them are cooked.

Water soluble vitamins include C and B complex. Water soluble vitamins are not stored in the body so are required on a daily basis. These vitamins can be destroyed by heat, exposure to air or lost in water used for cooking[4].

Minerals include **calcium, iron, zinc** and **magnesium.**

We often hear the word **metabolism** being bandied about which is the process your body converts what you eat and drink into energy and in turn the amount of calories you burn at rest[5]. Many people blame weight gain and inability to shed weight on a slow metabolism. Although our basic metabolic rate is determined by genetics, the foods we eat are usually the main driver of its efficiency level and any resulting weight gain.

A selection of nutrients including potential sources are detailed below[6,7].

Compound	Weight loss aid	Sources*
Vitamins		
Vitamin B-complex B2 B3 (Niacin) B6 B9 (Folate) B12	Supports and improves metabolism. Ensures a healthy thyroid	Meat, liver, fish, cheese, egg, whole grains, green leafy vegetables, broccoli, beans and oats
Vitamin C	Helps the body convert glucose into energy instead of being stored as fat	Sweet and chilli peppers, dark leafy greens, cabbage, broccoli, berries, kiwis and oranges
Vitamin D	Triggers weight loss primarily around the belly	Oily fish, eggs and about 20 minutes sun exposure daily
Choline and inositol	Breaks down fat preventing it from being deposited around the body	Liver, steak, eggs, wheat germ, nuts, cabbage, dark leafy greens including kale
Minerals		
Chromium Selenium Iodine Iron Zinc	Enhances fat burning process, improves sluggish thyroid gland, suppresses hunger pangs and food cravings	Liver, oily fish such as sardines and salmon, kelp, steak, beans & lentils, cheese, pumpkin seeds, brazil nuts, egg, spinach, onions and bananas
Other nutrients		
Omega-3 Omega-6 Amino acids Co-enzyme Q10	Helps reduce body fat by taking fat from fat cells and transporting it to muscle tissues to be used as energy and speed up fat metabolism	Meat, oily fish, mixed seeds including flax seeds, eggs, milk and avocados

If you eat fish and meat, a balanced, healthy diet should include at least two portions of fish a week including 1 portion of oily fish (around 140g per portion) – women no more than 2 portions of oily fish a week if pregnant, may become pregnant in future or currently breastfeeding, men up to 4 portions of oily fish per week[8]. Eat liver no more than once a week. However, if pregnant or taking vitamin supplements you should consult your doctor before eating liver[9]. Eat no more than 70g (2.5oz) a day of red meat which is equivalent to 2 standard beefburgers[10].

Nutrient content example of edamame beans and shortbread biscuits[11,12]

Macronutrients		Edamame (Soya) Beans (1 cup) 155g	% of RDA	2 Shortbread Biscuits (35g)	% of RDA
Water	g	112.8		1.3	
Energy	kcal	189		180	
Protein	g	16.86		1.88	
Fat	g	8.06		9.18	
Carbohydrate	g	15.41		22.32	
Fiber	g	8.1		0.5	
Sugars	g	3.4		7.6	
Micronutrients					
Minerals					
Calcium	mg	98	12%	5	1%
Iron	mg	3.52	25%	1.04	7%
Magnesium	mg	99	26%	5	1%
Phosphorus	mg	262	37%	23	3%
Potassium	mg	676	34%	31	2%
Sodium	mg	9		124	
Zinc	mg	2.12	21%	0.17	2%
Vitamins					
Vitamin C	mg	9.5	12%		
Vitamin B1 (Thiamin)	mg	0.31	28%	0.12	11%
Vitamin B2 (Riboflavin)	mg	0.24	17%	0.11	8%
Vitamin B3 (Niacin)	mg	1.418	9%	1.146	7%
Vitamin B6 (Pyridoxine)	mg	0.155	11%	0.025	2%
Vitamin B9 (Folate)	µg	482	241%	43	22%
Vitamin E	mg	1.05	9%	0.85	7%
Vitamin K	µg	41.4	55%	3.8	5%

It's advisable to restrict soya intake to no more than four servings per week.

I'm sure it's already clear that edamame beans are more nutritious for your cells, but it's worth considering the difference one food choice can make to your daily nutrient intake – "snack foods" should be an occasional treat and not a replacement for proper food.

In essence, simply restricting calories may not give you long-lasting weight loss. If the calories you consume lack necessary vitamins and minerals to stoke your metabolism, suppress cravings and in turn help your body burn fat, you may manage to lose weight in the short-term, but, in the long run, deficiencies in nutrients will royally screw up your metabolism leaving you with low energy levels and more inclined to overeat as your cells are screaming out to be fed. It's ironic but eating less food can eventually make you overweight and undernourished if it lacks sufficient nutrients.

One of the classic mistakes many of us make is to consume snacks low in nutrients and skip a proper meal to compensate which is not only counterproductive to weight loss, it can also be detrimental to your health – plus it will age you before your time, and no one wants that!

Signs of nutrient deficiency

The list of micronutrient deficiency signs is long; however, a few indications are tabled below.

Compound	Signs of deficiency
Vitamin	
Vitamin B-complex B2 B3 (Niacin) B6 B9 (Folate) B12	Fatigue, anxiety, depression, headaches, weakness and muscle pains/cramps, muscle tremors, tingling hands and feet, irritability, numbness and prickling in legs, water retention, nausea and stomach pains, poor concentration, poor memory, itchy eyes, sensitive to bright lights, eczema, mouth ulcers, cold sores, premature greying, hair loss or poor hair condition
Vitamin C	Bleeding gums, aches and pains, frequent colds and infections, nosebleeds
Vitamin D	Vitamin D controls calcium absorption – deficiency signs include backache and tooth decay
Choline and inositol	Eczema, frequent coughs and colds, nervousness, poor memory, high blood pressure
Minerals	
Chromium Selenium Iodine Iron Zinc	Sugar cravings, irritability after long gaps between meals, excessive thirst, hot and cold sweats, swollen thyroid gland in the neck, tiredness, poor concentration and memory, cold hands and feet, sleeplessness, itchiness, dandruff, high blood pressure, eczema, acne and psoriasis
Other nutrients	
Omega-3 Omega-6 Amino acids Co-enzyme Q10	Dry skin, frequent infections, poor co-ordination, memory and concentration problems, high blood pressure, inflammatory diseases such as rheumatoid arthritis, eczema and psoriasis, fatigue, obesity

I've never been one for counting calories – too cumbersome for me – but if and when I do, I will focus on **counting macronutrients** to ensure a balanced diet including sufficient intake of micronutrients. If you focus on eating minimally processed "real foods" close to their natural state, you'll be amazed how much you can eat and what each food group offers:

- **Carbs:** source of energy and micronutrients – fruits, vegetables, pulses and whole grains.
- **Protein:** repairs cells, involved in hormone production, forming antibodies to support immune function and creating enzymes – meat, poultry, fish, pulses, dairy, nuts and seeds.
- **Fats:** source of energy, maintain healthy cells, support hormone production and required to absorb fat soluble vitamins – oily fish, nuts, seeds, avocados, coconut/olive oil.

A typical western diet usually contains about 55% of calories from carbs, 23% protein and 22% fat. However, 40% carbs, 30% protein and 30% fat is believed to yield positive weight loss results.

Hints and tips on how to enhance nutrient absorption and avoid nutrient loss

Digestion starts in the mouth
Our digestive system, including enzymes, which facilitate breaking down food and absorbing nutrients starts in the mouth. With the help of teeth (physical) and saliva (chemical), the act of chewing kick-starts the digestive process. If you have a habit of eating fast and swallowing chunks of food, parts of your meal may pass through your body undigested with nutrients unabsorbed. Chewing food thoroughly will help maximise nutrient absorption.

Juicing vegetables
I've always struggled to eat enough veg – to this day I can't bear the thought of brussels sprouts! Vegetable juice is packed with bio-available (easy to digest) micronutrients. If your digestive system has been impaired by consuming too many processed and refined foods, your body may not

be able to absorb nutrients effectively: juicing is a great way to up your nutrient intake. The juice of one apple (or other fruit) can be added to make it more palatable if you struggle with the taste of vegetable juice on its own. I prefer to consume minimal juiced fruit opting to blend or eat fruit whole to retain fibre content and limit sugars.

The power of raw
Almost all foods that are packaged in boxes, cans or bags are processed to some extent and have been through a mechanical or chemical procedure to change or preserve it which can result in reduced nutrient content.

If, growing up, your household was anything like mine – where veg were cooked to death – seeing raw vegetables as a dish in their own right may have never been on the agenda. It's all too easy to obliterate food in the microwave or at high temperatures on the cooker. The more we mess about with our food, the less chance it has of retaining nutrients which can leave meals high in calories but low in nutritional value – some refer to this as **"empty calories"**. Eating raw foods is an essential part of a healthy diet. Adding raw vegetable dishes to your snacks and meal repertoire can help boost the amount of nutrients you consume. A 5 a day salad is a great way to incorporate raw foods (see page 87). It's worth noting that some foods will allow better absorption of specific nutrients when cooked e.g. lycopene found in tomatoes, an antioxidant, is easier for the body to absorb when cooked, so both raw and cooked veg is a good balance.

Be aware of anti-nutrients

Anti-nutrients are natural or synthetic substances that inhibit the body's ability to absorb or use nutrients. Plant based anti-nutrients are thought to be natural protection against insects – good for plants, not so good for us – as they can interfere with nutrient absorption in many ways like bind to other nutrients making them unavailable to the body, impair digestive enzymes, cause nutrients to be excreted or create a greater need for certain nutrients.

Examples of anti-nutrients and foods that may contain them

Anti-nutrient	Found in	How it impacts your body	Ways to reduce effect
Phytic acid	Whole grains including wheat and brown rice, nuts, seeds and beans	Can bind to essential minerals such as iron, zinc, calcium, and magnesium in the gut – linked to tooth decay/cavities	Soak whole grains and dry beans overnight (or quick soak dry beans*), fermenting/sprouting. Soak raw nuts/seeds in water for 4–9 hours
Oxalic acid	Spinach, cassava, beet and cocoa beans	Binds to iron and calcium reducing absorption	Consume with foods high in vitamin C and ensure sufficient vitamin D intake
Lectin	Beans, peas, lentils and whole grains	Can cause inflammation in the gut – linked to leaky gut syndrome	Soak in water for 4–24 hours. Never eat undercooked beans
Glucosino-lates	The list is long but includes cruciferous vegetables such as broccoli, kale and cabbage	Forms a substance called goitrin that can suppress the function of the thyroid gland by interfering with iodine uptake	Cooking – blanch, sauté, steam, shallow boil, or ferment. Rotate food choices. Eat iodine rich foods such as seaweed, seafood and eggs
Caffeine	Coffee and some soft drinks	Decreases ability to absorb zinc and some B vitamins. Also affects the liver by reducing vitamin A storage	Limit consumption. Up to 400mg of caffeine is considered safe for adults (which is about 4 cups of standard coffee)[13]
Other	Antibiotics and artificial sweeteners (found in sugar free drinks & chewing gum)	Can destroy good gut bacteria that aids digestion which can reduce nutrient absorption	Minimise and counteract with probiotics and fermented foods/unsweetened fermented drinks that contain good bacteria

* boil for 2 minutes in plenty of water, let stand for 1 hour then rinse and cook until soft.
** discard nuts that float to the top after being soaked as they may be damaged.

This by no means suggests that general consumption of food listed above is bad for you. Cruciferous vegetables, leafy greens and pulses are an essential part of a healthy diet. For every nutrient lost, your body will be provided with many others. However, overconsumption of any one food can reduce absorption of specific nutrients. Unless you are guzzling copious amounts of juiced kale, have a confirmed nutrient deficiency, experiencing signs of nutrient deficiencies or have digestive problems, it should not be a cause for concern.

The main point to take away here is to limit and avoid anti-nutrients where possible, particularly those that are synthetic (man-made), have a varied diet and rotate food choices to prevent deficiencies especially if juicing vegetables daily which can result in consuming several servings of veg in one sitting. Opt for mixed vegetable juice instead of single vegetable juices.

Consider going organic

A landmark paper published in the *British Journal of Nutrition* concluded that there are significant differences in the nutritional content of organic and non-organic crops[14]. Organic food contains substantially higher antioxidants – between 19% and 69% more than non-organic conventional food. Researchers suggest that switching to organic fruit and vegetables could give the same benefit as adding one or two portions of the recommended 5 a day[15].

Consider supplementation

Multivitamins: Ideally, we should get all nutrients required from a varied diet as the best sources of vitamins and minerals are from the food we eat. However, we all know how hard this can be plus, the foods we eat today contain fewer nutrients than food available 30–50 years ago. A report in the *Journal of Complementary Medicine* in 2001 highlights that US and UK Government statistics show a decline in trace minerals of up to 76% in fruit and vegetables over the period 1940–1991[16]. If you decide to take a vitamin supplement, try to opt for a food based non-synthetic multivitamin and be mindful that megadoses of some vitamins can be toxic, especially fat soluble vitamins which are stored in the body, so stick to one set to avoid overlapping. Also, we need to remember that vitamins are a supplement not replacement for food, so it is still important to eat a varied balanced diet.

Probiotics: Our digestive system is home to about 100 trillion bacteria – with the ideal ratio between good and bad bacteria in the gut being 85% good and 15% bad. Good bacteria (such as *lactobacillus acidophilus* and *lactobacillus rhamnosus*) help to digest food and absorb vitamins and minerals. Certain bad bacteria can contribute to obesity and make weight loss difficult. Studies have found that obese people had around 20% more bad bacteria and almost 90% less good bacteria than lean people[17].

Fat trap fact 2
All calories are not equal. Avoid "empty" calories and opt for nutrient dense foods. Prepare meals with nutrient retention in mind.

Chapter 4

Exercise

Weight loss without exercise is like going into a kick-boxing match with one hand tied behind your back – it's probably not going to end well. As one of my gym instructors used to say, "If you want to burn fat, you need to heat it up!"

Exercise definitely deserves its place in an effective weight loss programme and brings a whole host of other health benefits. However, it's not uncommon for people to exercise with the intention of losing weight but actually end up gaining weight. I will never forget the time I started jogging weekly with a friend and somehow managed to consistently put on weight week after week despite trying to cut back on food – if I hadn't been trying so hard I might have found it funny. It took some time for the penny to drop before I realised that my sugar intake was slowly increasing despite eating less food.

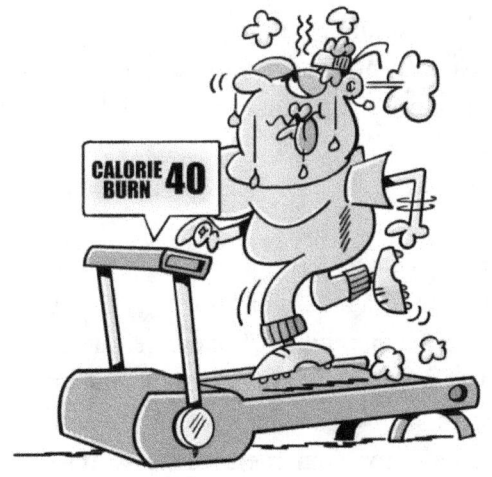

Studies show that people who start a new exercise programme can subconsciously eat more calories, partly because of the "I've just worked out so I deserve to splurge on food" mentality, and partly because exercise actually stimulates your appetite. So it's important to keep tabs on food intake even if you exercise regularly.

If you've ever slogged your guts out on a machine in the gym that monitors calories burned, you will already know that it takes shedloads of effort to burn off even 40 calories which, incidentally, is the approximate calorie content of half a shortbread biscuit. This is why your diet is paramount as it's generally easier to reduce the energy you take in than it is to burn it off, but, if you choose the right type of exercise, it can send calorie burn into overdrive.

At one point I acquired the nickname "cardio queen" because of my love of cardio-type classes, seeking out the hardest, lung-burning classes I could find – living by the mantra – go hard or go home! Back then it seemed to make sense. After all, I thought cardio was the best form of exercise to burn fat. But I was wrong. Although any exercise you enjoy and maintain on a regular basis will be of benefit, some forms of exercise can help you burn fat considerably faster than others. Limiting your exercise routine to cardio sessions is not the best approach to shift the weight.

Steady pace cardio such as jogging is more likely to use fat stores as a source of energy, but interval start-and-stop exercise such as circuit training, spinning, interval sprints and weightlifting will help you build muscle and increase your metabolic rate after exercise causing you to burn more calories for hours and possibly days after. This is referred to as the **"after-burn"** effect also known as "excess post-exercise oxygen consumption".

Although nearly all types of exercise will generate some after-burn, it is minimal for standard cardio. There's a strong correlation between number of calories burned post-exercise and intensity of activity. According to Victor Zammit, professor of metabolic biochemistry at Warwick University, "when your body is pushed during exercise, it can take up to three days for your metabolism to return to 'normal'." You know when you're breathing hard – trying to catch your breath during exercise? You have effectively created an **"oxygen-debt"**, one that your body will have to work to repay and refuel cells with energy. The more intense the exercise, the more oxygen the body requires after to make up for what it didn't have during exercise. This results in sustained **higher metabolic**

rate and in turn more calories burned. Just 20 minutes of high-intensity exercise is enough to increase calorie burn by up to 10%[18].

As if the after-burn effect wasn't a compelling enough reason for you to grab your trainers and sprint up the nearest hill.
A study published in 2007 compared short interval training against longer cardio sessions for fat loss. Professor Boutcher (Director of Fat Loss Laboratory, Faculty of Medicine, UNSW) took 45 overweight women, who maintained their usual eating habits, separating them into two groups. For 15 weeks, **Group 1** performed three 20-minute interval training workouts on a bike – 8 second sprints followed by 12 seconds of slow peddling (recovery) repeated for 20 minutes. **Group 2** performed 40 minutes of continuous steady pace cycling; both groups worked out 3 times a week on stationary bikes. **Group 1** (interval trainers) lost a significant amount of fat from their legs, buttocks and belly (average 3.9kg/8.6lbs lost). However, **Group 2** (steady cardio) didn't lose any fat at all despite exercising twice as long! In fact, women from **Group 2** increased body fat slightly by 0.5kg/1.1lb[19,20].

High-Intensity Interval training (HIIT) encourages short bursts of hormones, glucagon and adrenalin (epinephrine) which promotes the breakdown of fat from fat cells released into the bloodstream to be used as energy. HIIT also recruits both fast twitch muscles (which have a greater capacity for growth) and slow twitch muscles whereas steady pace cardio sessions mainly recruit slow twitch muscles (slow twitch muscles can be encouraged to grow through super slow reps with weights). Endurance exercise such as jogging is usually completed over the same distance each time, and generally at a similar pace so the body can adjust quickly and become efficient at saving energy. Steady pace exercise also encourages sustained release of stress hormones over long periods which can actually encourage fat accumulation.

HIIT can be hard on the body and amplify areas of weakness and imbalances increasing risk of injury. If your muscles are not strong enough to support each exercise, your joints and skeletal frame will bear the burden so it's important to prepare your body with a few weeks of general exercise first to build up fitness and strength particularly around joints to decrease the risk of injury. Ensure you eat balanced, nutritious meals, stretch regularly, allow yourself enough time to rest and drink sufficient water.

Not only are regular long cardio sessions less effective at burning fat over time, excessive long sessions can cause muscle wastage – think of the difference in muscle mass of a long distance runner verses that of a sprinter.

Muscle burns more calories than fat even when you're resting.
One pound of muscle can burn up to 10 calories per day, while 1 pound of fat can burn up to 3 calories a day[21]. The more muscle you have, the more calories you burn.

The amount of muscle you can gain will vary and depend on your workout, diet, genetics and muscle memory amongst other things. Realistically, unless you're racking up weights with the best of them, on average you can expect to build somewhere between 0.5–2 pounds of muscle in a month[22].

If you manage to gain 4lbs of muscle in 3 months, you can burn up to 40 calories more per day at rest which equates to 280 extra calories burned per week. Now you might be thinking for that amount of calorie burn it's hardly worth the effort, but you will also benefit from calories burned during the workout and the after-burn effect – not to mention being the proud owner of a tighter, fitter and more toned physique. Plus, working on building muscle can help counteract the effects of age-related sarcopenia which is the gradual loss of skeletal muscle mass after the age of 30. And there's more…

Muscle is a better place to store sugar than your gut
Carbohydrates (sugars) are broken down into glucose. If energy is not required immediately or you consume too much in one sitting, glucose will be stored as glycogen in the liver and muscle cells to be used later. When the liver and muscles have reached glycogen storage capacity, the remaining glucose will be converted and stored as fat, usually around the

midriff. The more muscle you have, the more capacity you have to store glucose as glycogen instead of fat.

An important part of building muscle is to feed muscle cells. Eating sufficient **protein** is the foundation of muscle growth. In the absence of sufficient dietary protein, our body will cannibalise (break down) muscle and other protein rich fibres such as ligaments and tendons to tap into protein stores to maintain bodily functions which will reduce muscle mass (see page 80 for suggested protein intake)[23].

I know some ladies are concerned about becoming too bulky but you don't need to worry as it takes a lot more effort than most people realise to gain masses of muscle, and you can always cut back on your routine if you don't like what you see. More muscle, faster results.

When we digest food, particularly carbs, a hormone, insulin, is released by the pancreas into the bloodstream. Insulin is a signal for cells to store glucose and other nutrients. Due to hormonal imbalances or genetics, sometimes cells do not respond to insulin properly and can become less efficient at receiving glucose resulting in low insulin sensitivity or **insulin resistance**. This is one of the reasons why some people can put in hours at the gym but see little or no change in muscle mass or tone as muscle will not grow properly without nutrients no matter how hard you workout.

Tips to improve insulin sensitivity
- Restrict refined sugars which enter the bloodstream fast and can cause extreme elevations in blood glucose
- Consume high fibre/low glycaemic load foods (see page 47)
- Regular exercise including HIIT can help improve insulin sensitivity[24]
- Drink green tea which can improve both insulin sensitivity and glucose tolerance[25]
- Eat omega-3 fatty acids – oily fish/fish oils, flax seeds/flax seed oil[26]
- Get sufficient sleep, reduce and manage stress levels[27]

When exercise becomes counterproductive

I'm lucky enough to genuinely enjoy exercise, but it never occurred to me that sometimes less can be more. There's a fine line between **training hard** and **overtraining**. It's important to understand that muscle does not grow during your workout, and intense exercise usually breaks down muscle. Muscle growth happens after exercise when the body is recuperating so we need enough time to rest[28]. Also, if you exercise too much or for too long, it can cause stress to the body and trigger high levels of a hormone called **cortisol.** The presence of cortisol results in enzymes breaking down protein and can encourage muscle wastage. Although there does need to be regular progression to continue to see results and avoid plateauing, you don't need to feel incapacitated for a week after exercising to have trained hard.

How much exercise is too much will vary from person to person. The right amount of exercise for you will depend on what your body is accustomed to and your diet. A good way to gauge your threshold is to assess how you feel post-workout, and on a day to day basis.

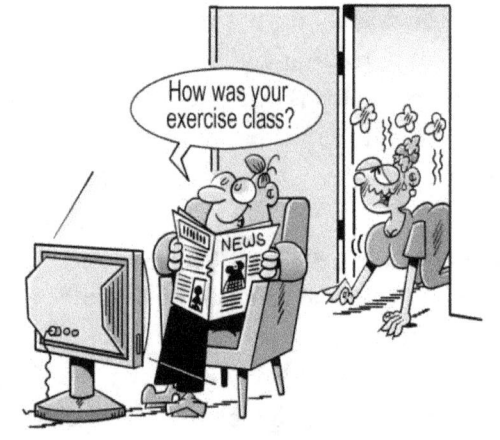

How was your exercise class?

NEWS

Signs of overtraining

- Your muscles ache way too much after your workout and the thought of squatting onto a toilet or walking down a flight of stairs fills you with genuine fear
- Frequent colds/regularly falling ill
- Painful joints and/or limbs
- Overly fatigued all the time
- Restlessness/unable to sleep
- Muscle loss/stop seeing results
- Can't be bothered to go to your next workout session

How to help readdress the balance

- **Eat plenty of mixed non-starchy vegetables.** Requirements for antioxidants increase post-exercise as physical activity increases free-radicals which can weaken your immune system. Vegetables, packed with nutrients and antioxidants, can help combat this.
- **Omega-3** – anti-inflammatory and support joints – oily fish, fish oil, flax seed, flax seed oil.
- **Eat a combination of carbs and protein post-workout** – essential to replenish and rebuild muscle, reduce muscle soreness, support immune function and suppress the release of cortisol which can rise sharply during intense or long exercise sessions
- **Avoid exercising at high intensity more than 2 days in a row.**
- **Consider reducing frequency, intensity or length of workouts.**
- **Get sufficient rest and sleep** – have at least one day off from strenuous exercise and maximise human growth hormone which rises during sleep and can help muscle growth[29].
- **Mix up your workouts** and incorporate at least one stretch or relaxation session to help reduce stress levels, keep muscles supple and prevent injuries.
- **Stretch all major muscle groups after every exercise session**.

I must admit I struggled with the concept of working out less to achieve better results, but if you are overtraining, taking your foot off the pedal on the exercise front can actually give you your biggest exercise breakthrough. However, for most of us, at some point in our lives, we need to focus on being more active.

Many people put exercise on a back burner due to low energy or lack of time, but if you commit to being more active and exercise regularly it can help boost energy levels making you more alert and improve productivity helping you free up more time.

Aim for 1–6 exercise sessions per week (including warm up and warm down).

Example of exercise routine:
- 1–3 HIIT/Interval training: 20–30 minutes – sprints / boxing / kick-boxing / spinning / elliptical / skipping / stair walking / circuits / strength training
- 1–3 Strength training: 20–60 minutes – circuits / body weight exercises / power yoga / weights
- 1 Low to medium steady pace cardio: 30–60 minutes – swimming / walking / jogging
- 1–2 Stretch/relaxation: 30–60 minutes – walking / meditation / t'ai chi / pilates / yoga

Adding resistance or weights into your exercise routine can be done using sandbags, vipers, kettle bells, medicine balls, weighted vests, standard bar and dumbbells, or incorporating body weight exercises, all of which can add variety.

It's best to exercise under the watchful eye of a qualified personal trainer or fitness instructor, especially when using weights or if you are new to regular exercise, which will help you get the most out of your sessions while having good form to avoid injuries. Alternatively, start with gentle exercise and progress slowly.

If you can't or simply don't enjoy exercise and sports, or even if you do, you can aim to be more active in your day to day life. Making a conscious effort to walk up escalators, take the stairs instead of using a lift, walk to the shops more or even complete the last leg of your commute on foot is an effective way to get into shape. Purchase a basic pedometer and aim to take a minimum of 10,000 steps a day – you'll be amazed by how much your fitness level can improve by increasing day to day activities.

Some gym classes are still an hour long which is fine if you enjoy it but you don't need to exercise for an hour to get results unless you want to, 20–30 minutes exercise sessions can be sufficient, but you will need to challenge yourself for the duration. If you can have a leisurely conversation during your peak exercise you are probably not pushing yourself hard enough.

Exercise tip
A short exercise session first thing in the morning on an empty stomach is more likely to tap into fat reserves as nutrients in the blood are depleted overnight and the body is forced to use stored fat as energy.

<u>Fat trap fact 3</u>
Muscle will help speed up your metabolism. 20–30 minutes of start-and-stop exercise can help blitz stubborn excess fat especially around your midriff.

Chapter 5

It's not me, it's my hormones

While you were sleeping

With countless growing demands, cutting back on sleep seems to be a logical solution, but is it? I've always believed that sleep can be so underrated and according to Professor Russell Foster (head of the Sleep and Circadian Neuroscience Institute at the University of Oxford), sleep is "the single most important health behaviour we have." Anyone who knows me is aware of my deep appreciation for slumber and it seems the phrase, "you snooze, you lose" can be quite apt when it comes to weight loss. While we are asleep, our mind and body is at work, growing and repairing cells and releasing hormones. Sleep is restorative. Two hormones which impact weight released during sleep are **ghrelin** and **leptin**.

Ghrelin – "hunger hormone" – released from the stomach, interacts with the brain to increase appetite, slow down your metabolism and decrease your body's ability to burn fat. Ghrelin also tends to encourage fat storage around the abdomen.

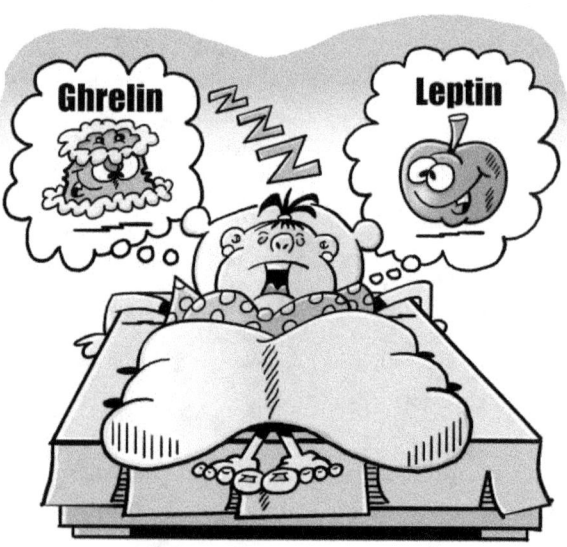

Leptin – "appetite suppressor hormone" – produced in fat cells, is the opposite hormone to ghrelin. Leptin helps regulate body weight by sending signals to the brain to reduce appetite and burn fat; the more fat you have, the more leptin you produce, unless you accumulate too much fat where sustained high levels of leptin can become ineffective as signals stop working, so the brain thinks there is a shortage of energy when there isn't[30].

If you don't sleep enough leptin levels can fall, leaving you unsatisfied after meals. Lack of sleep also causes ghrelin levels to rise, stimulating your appetite and making you crave more food. Not only does lack of sleep stimulate appetite in general, you are more likely to crave high-carb, fatty foods which tend to provide energy fast. Basically, if you don't sleep enough, you are more likely to binge on unhealthy food. Most experts agree, on average, adults need between 7–9 hours of sleep each night, and many of us fall short of the minimum on a regular basis[31]. I don't know about you, but a good day for me usually starts with a good night's sleep. If I don't sleep well enough, it's pretty much a struggle all day on many aspects including food. In addition to getting enough hours of sleep, if you generally wake up feeling tired and lethargic, you may not be getting enough quality sleep. Ask yourself soon after waking, do I feel well rested and refreshed?

Tips on improving quality of sleep

- **Calcium** – found in dairy products, sardines and sprats – is an effective natural sleep aid which supports production of sleep-inducing melatonin. Vitamin D intake is necessary to help absorb calcium.
- **Magnesium** – "nature's tranquiliser". Insufficient magnesium intake can result in sleep problems. Nuts, whole grains and dark leafy greens are rich sources.
- **Insomnia can be a symptom of vitamin B deficiencies** – particularly B1 and B5. Oily fish, lean pork, mushrooms, seeds, nuts, pulses and avocados are rich sources.
- **Avoid taking vitamins late at night** as some can have a stimulating effect.
- **Drink camomile tea** within an hour of going to bed to promote sleep.
- **Regular exercise**, particularly strength training, can promote sleep but avoid intense exercise within 3 hours of sleep[32]. A short walk before bed can also help induce sleep.

- **Unplug electrical equipment and switch off mobile phones** in the bedroom as they emit electromagnetic and radio frequency energy which can interfere with sleep.
- **Use a battery-powered alarm clock with a thermometer** and identify what room temperature works for you, taking into account changes in bedding and clothing.
- **Avoid using computers and gadgets,** which can stimulate your mind, 20 minutes before going to bed.
- **Eat your last meal at least 2 hours before going to bed** to allow proper digestion or have mainly non-starchy veg if eating late at night.
- **Consume sufficient carbs for you** – insufficient carb intake can trigger the release of adrenalin causing you to wake up abruptly in the middle of the night due to low blood sugar level. In general, you need to eat well to sleep well.
- **Avoid caffeinated and sugary foods/drinks late at night** which can act as stimulants. Drinking too much alcohol can also disrupt sleep.
- **Avoid lying in bed awake** which can cause anxiety and contribute to insomnia.
- **Sleep in a quiet, dark room** – street lights can trick your brain into thinking its daytime. Use blackout curtains – eye shades and foam ear plugs are alternatives.
- **Music** can have a profound effect on emotions, relaxing the mind, slowing down heart rate, decreasing stress hormones – search the web for music to promote sleep.
- **Place a drop of lavender essential oil** on the head of your mattress to help you relax.
- **Get at least 20 minutes of sun/daylight exposure everyday** and keep to regular sleep patterns to stay in sync with your natural sleep cycle, ideally go to bed before midnight.

Sleep and **stress** are interlinked – the more sleep you have, the less stressful everyday pressures can seem, and the less stressed you are the better you will sleep.

The stress factor

One of the main reasons people accumulate fat around their waist is because of the hormone **cortisol** which helps our body deal with stress. An inbuilt fight – or flight – response in the face of perceived danger stimulates the release of "stress" hormones adrenalin and cortisol prompting your liver to release glycogen (sugar) into the bloodstream providing instant energy to either fight or run. Although some stress is good, more often than not, our stressors come from looming deadlines, rowdy kids or bumper to bumper traffic, and are experienced for longer periods of time with no physical activity to utilise released energy[33].

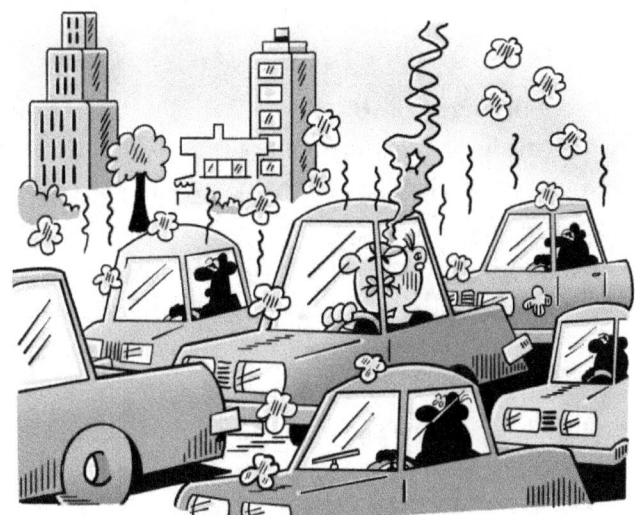

While cortisol levels remain high, your body ceases to burn fat as it thinks it needs to conserve energy. In the absence of physical activity, the body will store unused energy in a convenient place for fast access – as fat around your belly. In addition to this, high levels of cortisol sends signals to your brain to stimulate your appetite and stock up for more non-existent "battles" to come. Cortisol will tell your body to store fat. The effects of stress will vary from person to person and depend upon our individual coping mechanism and lifestyle – some of us are better at keeping calm when all is crumbling around us[34].

Signs of high stress levels:

- Poor memory.
- Loss of sense of humour.
- Irregular or absent periods.
- Feeling irritable/having mood swings.
- Teeth grinding or clenched teeth during sleep.
- Low immune system – frequent colds/infections.
- Muscle tension – particularly around shoulders.
- Increased appetite and cravings for "high-carb"/"high-fat" sugary foods.

Tips to help manage stress

- **Magnesium** helps calm nerves and is called upon during times of stress; sufficient magnesium intake can be effective at treating anxiety. Consider supplementing.
- **B vitamins** are known to have a positive effect on stress and anxiety.
- **A balanced diet** – essential to balance hormones and prevent nutrient deficiencies which can contribute to anxiety and stress.
- **Laughter** – and plenty of it – releases endorphins (happy hormones), stimulates organs and aids muscle relaxation.
- **Relaxing music** can help decrease stress levels (search the web for "RelaxDaily").
- **Reading** distracts the mind and can be relaxing.
- **Exercise** – walking/yoga/t'ai chi/meditation can help reduce cortisol levels.
- **Massage/acupuncture** increases blood circulation and relaxes muscles.
- **Take up a hobby**, watch a movie or indulge in TV.
- **Socialise** and connect with people (that don't stress you out).

Fat trap fact 4

Insufficient sleep and high levels of stress can lead to cravings and binge eating while preventing fat burn. Use suggested methods to improve sleep and try to manage stress.

Chapter 6

Toxic overload

For many, the term "**detox**" conjures up an image of someone righteously sipping on vegetable juice on top of a remote mountain. Although this approach to detox is effective, the process of detoxification can be far simpler and a lot closer to home. Detoxification is part of the body's everyday function, eliminating toxins or anything else the body doesn't want or need[19]. Toxins can be viewed in two main categories:

- **External** such as pesticides (used on crops) and BPA (bisphenol A – an industrial chemical used in some plastics and the lining of canned food and drinks).
- **Excessive internal inflammation** triggered by an imbalanced diet.

External toxins
BPA can leach into food and drinks from plastic bottles and the lining of cans. Substances used to produce some till and ATM receipts can be absorbed into the bloodstream, cosmetic and household products can contain unwanted substances, chemical residue from sprays find their way into the food chain, exhaust fumes, cigarette smoke, mercury, radiation, general pollution – the list goes on. There are a whole host of substances that can enter our system daily via the air we breathe, food we eat and products we use. Although the individual quantities used by manufacturers of some of these chemicals are not deemed to pose a health risk to the public, at best, the long-term effects of a combination of these substances from a weight loss perspective are unknown, but more likely; these compounds can mess with your hormones and affect weight loss efforts.

A programme conducted by the Environmental Protection Agency (EPA) analysed human fat samples looking for types of toxins that accumulate in fat in 1982 and 1987. Four industrial solvents and one dioxin – a toxic compound produced as a by-product in some manufacturing processes –

were found in all fat samples, highlighting the presence of toxins in body fat[35].

Excessive internal inflammation
Inflammation in the body helps us get rid of harmful viruses and bacteria and removes unwanted, damaged cells. This is followed by an anti-inflammatory response which kick-starts cell repair and healing. Both processes are necessary for health and wellbeing.

Inflammation is controlled by a group of hormones called eicosanoids and derived from the fat we eat. One essential fatty acid that can be made into eicosanoids is arachidonic acid (AA) – which is an omega-6 fatty acid. Although the body requires some AA to induce inflammation when needed, too much AA can put our immune system at risk and cause unwanted cellular damage – our diet can activate inflammation in the body. Food high in omega-6 including vegetable oils, margarine, certain farmed fish like tilapia and refined processed carbohydrates such as pastries and cakes (which often contain vegetable oils or margarine) are linked to increasing levels of AA in the body[36]. Ultimately, omega-6 fats increases production of AA and is the building block of inflammation hormones, which in excess can be toxic and disrupt weight loss efforts.

Our body is doing us a favour
To prevent high levels of toxins in the bloodstream, which can harm vital organs, our body encapsulates toxins in fat and deposits them around the body, leaving the toxin dormant. If and when fat, which is holding onto toxins, is burned and used as energy, the toxins are released back into the bloodstream. If these toxins are not excreted from the body fast enough, to keep us safe, the body will remove the toxins from the blood and store them, once again, in fat cells. Fat burn without regular detoxification can lead to a cycle of your body trying desperately to reduce toxin levels in the blood by storing fat.

Given that over 140,000 substances, significantly more than predicted, have been pre-registered for commercial use with the European Chemicals Agency following EU's REACH* Regulation, I don't fancy your chances of living a chemical-free life unless you pack up and ship off to a deserted island somewhere – and even then you would probably stumble upon some toxic strain that's made its way to new pastures[37,38]. The way I see it, it's virtually impossible to avoid all toxins in the modern world, especially if you live in a city or anywhere remotely industrialised. Ingesting some toxins has just become part of the package and a price we pay for convenience.

Our body's attempt to remove toxins from the blood is one of the reasons why people tend to regain weight rapidly following a detox retreat in a much less polluted place, and why some of us feel a bit rough when attempting weight 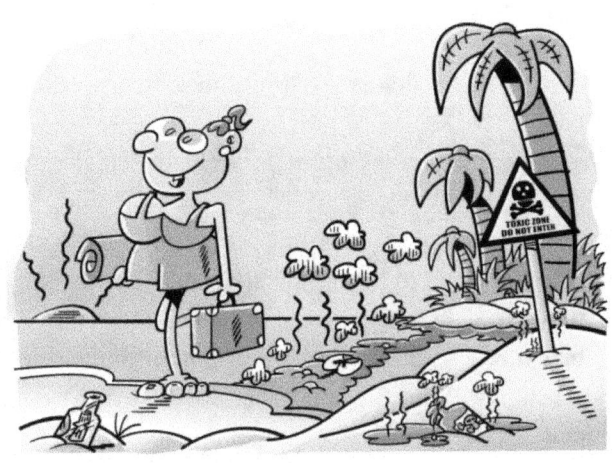 loss. With this in mind, the best approach is to try to minimise ingesting toxins (avoiding damaged cans, only reuse appropriate water bottles etc) and maximise the body's natural day to day toxin elimination process through **urination** and **bowel movements**[39].

Urination: Drink sufficient water throughout the day. Thirst and dark urine are signs of dehydration. Unless you are taking supplements such as B vitamins which can alter the colour, urine should be clear with a hint of yellow.

Bowel movements: Generally, up to 3 well-formed bowel movements a day is considered "normal". Bowel movements are one of the best ways to get toxins out of the body. To facilitate this, we need to eat enough fibre (at least 30 grams daily), from fruits and vegetables in addition to drinking enough water which will help move things along. On average, most people in the UK consume about 14 grams (US, 15 grams) of fibre a day, which is short of the minimum[40,41].

Fibre, particularly soluble fibre, is known to bind to toxins and as our body is unable to absorb fibre; both the toxin and fibre are excreted out of the body. Eating plenty of fibre rich foods should definitely be on the menu to help weight loss. Besides, constipation is no fun!

Constipation can be defined as infrequent bowel movements (3 times or less per week), the sensation of not emptying bowels or straining for more than 25% of the time when emptying bowels. One in 7 people suffer from constipation in the UK[42]. If you continue to struggle to get enough fibre in your diet, flax seeds or psyllium husk can be taken as a supplement.

Sweating, induced by regular exercise, can also help remove toxins.

Toxins accumulate in the body over time so the key to efficient detoxification is to keep your liver and kidneys in good working condition as they are responsible for identifying and removing toxins from the blood to be excreted. The liver can eliminate toxins released from fat if fat burn is gradual – about 2 pounds per week[43]. If fat is burned much faster than this, it is likely to trigger fat accumulation depending on levels of toxicity in fat cells.

Signs your liver may be overwhelmed or not functioning at its optimum
- Chronic fatigue.
- Bloating and gas.
- Trembling hands.
- Inability to lose weight.
- Acid reflux and heartburn.
- Itchy or oversensitive skin.
- Mood swings/anxiety/depression.
- Yellowish skin and/or eyes (symptom of jaundice).
- Forgetfulness, poor memory, confusion and drowsiness.
- Swollen abdomen (ascites), legs, ankles or feet (oedema) due to fluid build-up.

Ways to assist liver cleanse

Juicing vegetables is an effective way to help detoxify the body, packed with nutrients that activate and boost production of liver detoxifying enzymes. By juicing vegetables you can benefit from several servings of veg in one cup (note: vegetable juice counts for a maximum of one portion towards your 5 a day no matter how much you have[44]).

Raw fruit and veg can carry parasites and harmful bacteria from particles of soil and debris attached to crops that can't be seen with the naked eye. Although a healthy digestive system can eradicate most of these not everyone's digestive system is healthy, so it's important to wash fresh produce thoroughly including fruit that can transfer parasites onto flesh when being peeled. A solution of white vinegar and water can be used to remove certain pesticides and bacteria (up to 10% vinegar and the remainder water). Briefly soak fresh fruit and veg for a minute or so and rinse thoroughly (not appropriate for delicate food such as berries). Buying foods from your local farmers market is a good way to interact with farmers so you can ask what pesticides, if any, are used on crops.

Good hygiene while preparing and handling all raw food including meat, poultry and seafood will help prevent spreading bacteria to other foods and kitchen surfaces. Cooking meat, poultry and seafood at the recommended temperature and for suggested length of time can also help kill bacteria and parasites.

Go organic
More than 320 pesticides can be used routinely in non-organic farming, and many pesticides remain on food even after washing and cooking[45]. Organic farmers severely restrict the use of artificial chemical fertilisers and pesticides. As a result, pesticide residue on organic crops is significantly lower than non-organic crops. See a list of cleanest and dirtiest conventional fruits and vegetables at: http://www.ewg.org/foodnews. Organic free-range livestock and organic (wild) fish are also good food options as conventional meat and farmed fish can be routinely given antibiotics and grain/corn feed which can be

high in omega-6. As a result, livestock can also suffer from toxic fat or absorb contaminants from their environment which we then consume.

Foods to support liver and kidney cleanse and assist in detoxifying the body are listed below[46].

• Cruciferous vegetables* • Beets and carrots • Spinach • Garlic • Tomatoes	• Celery • Cucumbers • Parsley • Pumpkin • Onions	• Grapefruit • Watercress • Spices such as turmeric, and cinnamon • Algae: spirulina, chlorella

Such as broccoli, cauliflower, brussels sprouts, kale, pak choi and cabbage.

Supplements to support detoxification – 1 or 2 of the following for 2 weeks at a time:

Supplement	Daily intake	Benefits
Fresh lemon juice	1–2 lemons with hot water	Stimulates bile production to help flush out toxins
Dandelion tea	1–2 cups daily	Increases bile flow which breaks down fat
Burdock tea	1–2 cups daily	Enhances your body's efforts to get rid of toxins
Milk thistle extract	As directed	Relieves congestion of the liver and kidneys
Psyllium husk	As directed	Helps bowel movements and removal of toxins

Cleansing teas such as peppermint, nettle, fennel and camomile are also good for daily detox.

Balance omega-6 and omega-3 fatty acids. Bringing balance between omega-3 and 6 fatty acids consumed can help reduce levels of internal AA toxicity. The recommended ratio of omega 3 to omega 6 is around 1:3 (whereas the average UK diet has a ratio of 1:10 and the average US diet ranges between 1:20 to 1:50)[47,48]. Limiting omega-6 rich foods, including vegetable oils and margarine while increasing foods high in omega-3 such as oily fish (within guidelines), fish oil, flax seed oil and flax seeds, can help reduce excessive inflammation. Turmeric, ginger and rosemary also have anti-inflammatory properties[49].

Fat trap fact 5
When you think of weight loss, think of detox as its other half – they go hand in hand. Toxins can make your body hold onto fat with any weight loss being short-lived.

Chapter 7

Insulin and trapped fat

Fat-adapted or sugar-burner? If you happen to know someone who always seems to say "I haven't eaten all day" and is super slim, other than finding it slightly annoying, I'm sure you've wondered how it is even possible. The chances are he or she is most certainly "fat-adapted". When you are fat-adapted your body is efficient at burning stored and dietary fat for energy and is able to switch between burning sugars, when available, to burning stored fat when not. For those of us who mainly burn and are dependent on sugar, the body struggles to convert stored fat back into energy. In our hunter-gatherer days we would have all been fat-adapted but increased consumption of carbs, particularly refined carbs, has cultivated a reliance on sugar[50]. Fat stored around the belly is food (energy) saved for later which may or may not be nutrient dense but energy all the same. "Fat-burners" are less likely to feel hungry between meals as their body is efficient at tapping into fat stores in the absence of eating a meal, whereas "sugar-burners" are usually eager for their next food fix despite having ample stored fat.

Insulin is a hormone that regulates how the body uses and stores glucose. It helps control blood sugar (glucose) levels by signalling to the liver, muscle and fat cells to take energy in the form of glucose along with other nutrients from the blood to be used as fuel[51].

Blood glucose level rises in response to food we eat (particularly carbs). For reasons including diet – too many refined carbs and sugars – and genetics, insulin levels can spike up and remain higher than "optimal" range after meals. If insulin is released in large quantities repeatedly, receptors in muscle and liver cells can be damaged over time making them less sensitive to the presence of insulin in the blood which will restrict glucose uptake and glycogen storage. When our body is working as it should, fat cells would be called upon for energy on a regular basis and, in turn, fat accumulation would be low.

How digestion of carbs work

Eat carbs

⬇

Carbs are broken down and digested into glucose (sugar)

⬇

Glucose moves into bloodstream – the body detects an increase in blood sugar and sends signal to pancreas

⬇

Pancreas releases insulin (to transport energy to cells)

⬇

Bloodstream takes glucose and insulin to cells that need energy

⬇

Blood sugar level starts to fall

⬇

Remaining glucose converted and stored as fat

⬇

Fat stores used as energy between meals

Insulin resistance is a condition where the body does not respond properly to insulin, and glucose builds up in the blood instead of being absorbed by cells[52]. High blood sugar level then prompts the body to convert glucose and store as fat. Despite having generous fat stores, the presence of high insulin levels will inhibit fat being released from fat cells into the bloodstream to be used as energy (as insulin sends signals of energy storage, not energy release). High insulin levels create a cycle where the body stores fat with ease but is unable to release fat for energy. Some experts refer to this as the **"fat trap"**[53]. While insulin levels are high your body will not burn fat. Further to this, because energy is not being released from fat cells, the brain sends out hunger signals encouraging you to eat quick energy releasing foods so you are more likely to crave **high-carb/high-fat foods.**

Insulin resistance/low insulin sensitivity

Eat carbs

⬇

Carbs are broken down and digested into glucose (sugar)

⬇

Glucose moves into bloodstream – the body detects an increase in blood sugar and sends signal to pancreas

⬇

Pancreas releases insulin (to transport energy to cells)

⬇

Bloodstream takes glucose and insulin to cells but cells are less responsive to insulin and inefficient at taking in energy

⬇

Cells continue to send out signals for energy – liver releases stored glucose and pancreas releases more insulin to try to overcome resistance

⬇

Blood glucose levels continue to rise, sustained high blood sugar levels can be dangerous and harm vital organs so the body converts and stores as much glucose as it can as fat – fat cells generally continue to respond to insulin

⬇

The body struggles to tap into stored fat as insulin levels still remain high so cells continue to send out hunger signals

Sugar[54]

Sucrose, glucose and fructose are carbohydrates referred to as simple sugars and provide the same amount of energy but are used differently in the body.

Glucose – found in fruit and nearly all "carb foods" – is a monosaccharide meaning one sugar – the simplest carbohydrate molecule. Glucose is the most important sugar as all cells in the body can use it for energy. Our body can also produce glucose from protein or fat if needed.

Fructose – also found in fruit and added to food and drink – is a monosaccharide that is only used by the liver and not used as energy by muscle cells.

Sucrose – commonly known as table sugar – a disaccharide – one molecule of fructose and one molecule of glucose bound together. The body breaks down sucrose into glucose and fructose.

High fructose corn syrup (HFCS) is a man-made sweetener derived from corn and composed of fructose, glucose and other higher sugars. Studies confirm that sucrose (table sugar) and particularly fructose, can cause weight gain[56,55].

How sugar can make you fat fast

- Sugar is absorbed into the bloodstream fast, and if we eat too much of it, it can cause insulin levels to spike which will not only store unused energy as fat but, in excess, can also cause insulin resistance, creating the fat trap cycle.
- Sugar makes food more palatable encouraging you to eat more. I can't imagine getting excited about tucking into a tub of ice cream without sugar.
- Table (and added) sugar contain little or no vitamins, minerals, protein or fat, yet provides 16 calories in energy from every teaspoon, and is therefore empty calories.
- When we eat sugar (especially combined with fat) our brain releases dopamine, a hormone that can activate the pleasure-reward centre in our brain. If we associate pleasure with food it becomes moreish, so it's very easy to eat too much.

Why fructose is particularly fattening

- Unlike glucose, fructose does not stimulate production of leptin (appetite suppressant hormone) which can leave you unsatisfied. It's easy to eat or drink your way through 200–500 calories that contain fructose and still feel hungry or left wanting more.
- When we eat more fructose than the liver can use, the remainder will be converted and stored as fat. As the liver is the only organ that uses fructose it's easy to eat too much.
- When fructose is metabolised, it is the only sugar that generates uric acid (a waste compound found in the blood). Studies show that uric acid has a significant role in determining body weight and is a predictor of obesity[56,57]. High levels of uric acid is associated with increased risk of insulin resistance, Gout and other illnesses such as non-alcoholic fatty liver and high blood pressure (hypertension). It is for this reason that excess fructose can not only make you fat fast, but can also make you sick.

Although fruit (and some vegetables) contain fructose, fruit provides the body with a variety of important nutrients and therefore is an essential part of a balanced diet in moderation, particularly when consumed with its natural fibre content which slows down the absorption of fructose. Plus fruit in its natural state generally contains significantly less fructose than food and drinks with added sugar. Eating 2–3 portions of different fruit daily and plenty of mixed non-starchy vegetables will be beneficial for most people.

New guidelines from the World Health Organization suggest limiting intake of added sugar and sugars naturally present in honey, syrups and fruit juices, to avoid health issues, to 25 grams per day which is around **6 teaspoons** of sugar for an adult of normal Body Mass Index (BMI) down from 12 teaspoons or 50 grams. To give this some context, 1 tablespoon of ketchup contains around 1 teaspoon of sugar, and a can of sugar-sweetened soft drink can contain up to 10 teaspoons of sugar which would take you over the suggested daily limit[58].

You might think you don't consume a lot of sugar because you avoid sweets and don't add sugar when drinking tea, but if you eat packaged foods you'll be surprised at what lurks within from both added and natural sugars.

Natural and added sugar content of common snacks and foods in approximate equivalent teaspoons[59,60,61,62,63,64,65,66,67,68,69,70,71,72,73,74,75]

Food	Quantity	Tspn of sugar	Food	Quantity	Tspn of sugar
Cereal			**Biscuits**		
Alpen Original	6 tbsp (50g)	3	Chocolate digestive	2	2
Alpha Bites Multigrain	6 tbsp (25g)	1	Ginger nut	2	1
All Bran	6 tbsp (50g)	2	Jaffa cakes	2	3
Honey & Nut Clusters	6 tbsp (50g)	3	Custard cream	2	2
Shreddies	6 tbsp (50g)	2			
			Drinks		
Bread			Ginger ale	240 ml	5
Croissant	1 medium	2	Bitter lemon	240 ml	6
Brown/wholemeal	2 slices	1	Red Bull	250 ml can	7
			Sun exotic tropical fruit	288ml carton	8
Confectionary			Coca-Cola	330 ml can	8
Maltesers	1 bag (37g)	5	Mighty malt	330 ml bottle	11
Snickers bar	1 bar	6	Oasis (summer fruits)	500ml bottle	5
Mars bar	1 bar (36g)	5	This Juicy Water Lemon & Lime	420 ml bottle	9
Aero Bubbly	1 bar (40g)	6	Innocent Super Smoothie	360 ml bottle	10
Crunchie	1 bar (40g)	6	Ribena Blackcurrant	500ml bottle	12
KitKat	4 fingers	6	Pret freshly squeezed orange juice	500 ml bottle	12
Cadbury Dairy Milk Chocolate	1 bar (45g)	6	Starbucks signature hot chocolate	Venti - soy	13
Hard boiled sweets	per sweet	2	Eat mocha chiller	Large	22
Rowntree's Fruit pastilles	1 tube	3	Costa Ice – red berry cooler	Massimo	23
Milkybar Buttons	1 packet (30g)	4			
Smarties	Hexatube (38g)	6	**Cakes/desserts**		
Twix Twin	2 biscuits (50g)	6	Chocolate sponge cake	1 medium slice	6
Twirl	2 fingers (43g)	6	Doughnut	1 medium	3
Haribo (starmix)	mini bag (20g)	2	Sponge cake with icing	1 medium slice	11
Skittles	1 packet (55g)	12	Cupcake with icing	1 medium	6
Bassetts Murray Mints	per sweet	1	McDonalds strawberry sundae	1 container	11
Polo (original)	1 tube (34g)	8	McDonalds vanilla milkshake	medium	14
Nakd (cashew cookie)	Small bar	3			
The food doctor	Get Set Bar	4	**Yoghurt**		
Yoghurt coated peanuts & raisins	40g	5	Yoplait Light Yogurt (strawberry)	1 Container	2
Nutri-Grain Elevenses	1 bar	4	Frozen yoghurt (vanilla)	1/2 cup	4
Green & Black Creamy	100g bar	12			
			Soup		
Oatmeal			Tinned tomato	1/2 can	2
Quaker Instant Oatmeal Apple & Cinnamon	1 cup (43g)	3			
			Tinned veg		
			Heinz Beans	1/2 medium tin	2
Sauces/dressing			Sweet corn	1/2 medium tin	1
Honey BBQ sauce	2 tbsp	3			
Tomato ketchup	2 tbsp	2	**Takeaway**		
Thousand Island	2 tbsp	1	Chicken tikka masala	Typical portion	8
Salad cream	2 tbsp	1	Cantonese sweet and sour chicken	Typical portion	16

Shocked? I know I was. On average, adults in Western Europe consume 101 grams of sugar per day which is equal to 24 teaspoons of sugar[76]. Consider how much sugar you currently get through in one week.

When buying packaged foods, remember 4 grams of sugar is roughly equal to 1 teaspoon of sugar.

How do you know if you have insulin resistance or low insulin sensitivity?

Insulin resistance or low insulin sensitivity usually has no symptoms and can go undetected for several years but people with these conditions will generally have high levels of insulin throughout the day. Insulin resistance/low insulin sensitivity can be associated with:

- You seem to gain fat on a calorie-controlled diet but lose weight on a low-carb diet.
- You experience energy slumps within 60 minutes of eating a meal and generally feel lethargic.
- You feel ravenous if you miss a meal despite having ample belly fat.
- You are in the obese category of the BMI chart.
- You have abdominal obesity – high level of (visceral) fat around organs which is indicative of low insulin sensitivity[31]. Measurements to gauge excess abdominal fat:[77,78]
  - **Waist:** Men>102cm/40inches, Women>89cm/35inches
  - **Waist/hip ratio:** Men>1, Women>0.85 (waist/hip in inches)

As carbs are mainly responsible for increasing blood sugars and elevating insulin levels, insulin resistance or low insulin sensitivity is an indication that your diet is too sweet i.e. contains too much sugar/carbs for you based on various factors including your activity levels and general health. Over time, insulin resistance can develop into type 2 diabetes.

Dr Robert Lustig a paediatrician and author of *Fat Chance: the bitter truth about sugar* who specialises in treating overweight children and spent 16 years studying the effects of sugar on the body, blames insulin for 75–80% of all obesity and why many refer to insulin as our main "fat storing hormone"[79]. Improved insulin sensitivity can yield significant weight loss.

Two approaches can help improve insulin sensitivity:
1. Intermittent fasting
2. A low-carbohydrate diet without compromising the function of insulin

1. Intermittent fasting

Intermittent fasting can improve insulin sensitivity and modulate levels of visceral fat[80]. Fasting can either be done on one or two non-consecutive days similar to the 5:2 diet with two "fasting days" where daily calories are restricted (600: men, 500: women) or fasting overnight for 14–18 hours and restrict eating to a window of 7–8 hours during the day. The idea is that your body is forced to look for energy and tap into fat stores once nutrients in the blood have been depleted. Fasting results in less insulin (fat storing hormone) and more glucagon (fat releasing hormones) turning your body into fat burning mode. If you eat a lot of high-carb foods, are insulin resistant or simply do not eat enough nutritious foods, you may struggle to fast and suffer from low energy levels, especially at the beginning, as your body is less efficient at converting fat back into energy. So the focus should be on eating plenty of nutrient dense foods on both fasting and non-fasting days.

2. Low-carbohydrate diet

Farmers have known for thousands of years that carbs can help fatten cattle up fast which is one of the reasons why farmed animals are often fed grains or corn. If you've ever experienced that sleepy feeling after eating, it probably followed a meal high in carbs resulting in raised blood sugar level and a spike in insulin followed by a subsequent "sugar crash". There's no doubt that maintaining blood sugar levels within an "optimal" range and avoiding blood sugar highs and lows, is an effective way to lose weight. Carb foods are a good source of energy but we generally eat too much for our lifestyle and activity level. A low-carb diet can help reduce insulin levels and coax the body into burning fat – protein generally has a lesser impact and fat has no impact on insulin. Studies show that a low-carb diet is a fast and effective way to lose weight – monitoring carbs by grams can promote efficient weight loss.

Many foods contain carbs including fruit, cereals, bread, potatoes, pasta, vegetables, pulses, whole grains and dairy, but each food group and variation of food type will contain different quantities of carbs e.g. 100 grams of plain Greek yoghurt contains 3.6 grams of carbs whereas low-fat fruit yoghurt can contain up to 19 grams of carbs. One cup of cooked basmati rice provides 40 grams of carbs compared to short grain rice which provides 53 grams, while non-starchy vegetables generally contain minimal carbs, so it is possible to eat more carb foods but consume less total carbs.

Low carbs doesn't mean no carbs. If carb intake is too low for you, the function of insulin can be compromised. Depending on how reliant your body is on sugar, too little glucose from carbs can have an undesirable effect and some may experience symptoms including:

- Dizziness.
- Irritability.
- Tiredness/lethargy.
- Unable to focus/concentrate – "brain fog".
- Interrupted sleep/waking up abruptly in the middle of the night.

So the question is how low should you go? All carbs are not the same; needless to say, sugary, refined and processed carbs low in nutrients such as cakes and biscuits should be the first to go. In addition to this, consuming low glycemic index/low glycemic load carbs and monitoring your carb intake by grams can be beneficial.

Glycemic index (GI)/Glycemic load (GL).
Gone are the days of simply categorising carbs as complex being good and simple being bad as the focus now is more on how foods affect blood sugars. **GI** indicates how quickly carbs are digested, broken down and released into the bloodstream. High GI raises blood sugar more than medium or low GI which has a slower rate of digestion, whereas **GL** measures the amount of carbs in a standard serving of each food and rate of digestion. Foods with a GL under 10 are considered low and have a lesser impact on blood sugars assuming you eat the suggested serving size or less. GL of 11–20 is moderate impact with above 20 being high and likely to cause blood sugar spikes[81]. Although GI indicates how quickly carbs are absorbed, it is not necessarily based on how much we usually eat in one sitting which can impact changes in blood sugars e.g. a sweet is virtually all carbs and is absorbed quickly, but if we generally only eat one it is unlikely to impact blood sugar levels. Blood sugar is dependent on both speed of absorption and amount of carbs consumed in one sitting. GL is a good indicator as it takes into account both standard servings and impact on blood sugars.

Glycemic load of foods (different food brands can have different glycemic reading)[82,83,84]

Foods	Low glycemic load foods	High glycemic load foods
Fruit	Lemons, limes, passion fruit, grapefruit, avocados, strawberries and other berries, blackcurrants, cherries, melons, apples, pears, plums, mandarins, pomegranates	Raisins, dates, figs other dried fruit [ripe banana – moderate GL]
Non-starchy vegetables	Asparagus, carrots, peas, tomatoes, lettuce, cucumber, courgettes, peppers, mange tout, pumpkin, onions, squash, turnips, red cabbage, brussels sprouts, cauliflower, leafy greens (kale, spinach), celery, mushrooms, broccoli	
Root vegetables	New potato, sweet potato, yam, swede	Large floury white potatoes, French fries, mashed potato
Bread	Sourdough, rye, linseed, barley and granary, oat cakes, seeded breads, [pitta bread and rye crackers – moderate GL]	White/wholemeal bread, breadstick, cream crackers, bagels, West Indian raisin and hard dough bread
Cereal	Whole oats, traditional porridge, no added sugar muesli, semolina, quinoa, (plain instant oats and All Bran – moderate GL)	Sweetened cereals, rice based cereals, Bran Flakes, Shredded Wheat, wheat biscuits, Corn Flakes
Pasta / noodle	Egg-based pasta, mung bean noodles, buckwheat (soba) noodles, couscous (a type of pasta produced from wheat) [fettuccini pasta moderate – GL]	Pasta ready meals and overcooked pasta, spaghetti, macaroni [wholemeal pasta – moderate GL]
Rice	Long grain, wild, and basmati rice. Bulgur or cracked wheat, pearl barley	Short grain, sticky white rice, rice cakes
Snacks	Waffles, ice cream, plain popcorn, chocolate (3 small squares) based on some manufactures serving sizes	Sweet popcorn, yoghurt coated raisins, cakes with icing/filling, biscuits, sweetened soft drinks, pretzels, chocolate (in larger quantities)

Although raisins (like other dried fruit) will provide you with nutrients, up to 72% in weight is sugar[37], so from a weight loss perspective a small handful of raisins is like eating a small handful of sweets. Even if you do not eat much snack foods such as cakes and biscuits, you can still gain weight from eating too many other high GL foods such as whole wheat bread, pasta and some cereals.

Monitoring carbs by the gram – examples of carb intake by grams[85]

Slow but steady weight loss/maintenance – "moderate" carb intake throughout the week.
150–200 grams per day (600–800 calories)
- 5 a day salad and plenty of mixed non-starchy vegetables including soup.
- 1–3 portions of fruit: 1 portion (80g) is roughly 1 medium apple or 2 small fruits such as plums or satsumas[86].
- 1–2 portions of starch: sweet potatoes and healthier grains like quinoa and rice.
- 1 portion of pulses: 1 portion is roughly 3 heaped tablespoons.

Efficient and consistent weight loss – "low" carb intake for alternating days.
60–100 grams per day (240–400 calories)
- 5 a day salad and plenty of mixed non-starchy vegetables including soup (without potato).
- 1–2 portions of fruit.
- 1 portion of pulses.
- 1 portion of starch.

Fast weight loss – "very low" carb intake for 1 or 2 non-consecutive days a week.
50–60 grams per day (200–240 calories)
- 5 a day salad and plenty of mixed non-starchy vegetables including soup (without potato).
- 1 portion of lower carb starch like sweet potato.
- 1–2 portions of low-carb fruits: strawberries/avocado or 1 portion of pulses.

Fibre

Adding fibre to your meals lowers the glycemic load by slowing down the rate of digestion. High-fibre foods add bulk which makes you feel fuller for longer and tend to provide less energy which means fewer calories. Increased insoluble dietary fibre intake for 3 days will significantly improve insulin sensitivity[87]. Most fruit and veg are high in fibre. Split peas, green peas, lentils and black beans are fibre rich. Avocados and raspberries boast the most fibre in fruit followed by apples and pears, while artichoke and broccoli top the list for vegetables[88].

Fat trap fact 6

Sustained high blood sugar levels will keep you in fat storing mode. Control "fat storing hormone" insulin by restricting sugar and consuming low-carb/low-GL food.

Chapter 8

The good, the not so good, and the ugly

In the past, those seeking to lose weight were advised to steer clear of fat, with most dietary fats lumped into one box labelled "open with caution". In the early 1980s a number of articles linked increased dietary cholesterol with increased blood cholesterol. To simplify things, general advice to the public was to reduce overall fat consumption from our diet in a bid to improve health. This spawned the rise of low-fat diets. What nobody anticipated was that the food industry would substitute animal fats with vegetable fats or replace fats with sugar on such a major scale while keeping calorie content the same. Over the following two decades, experts observed, while consumption of dietary fat reduced, obesity rates increased.

Why I try to avoid vegetable oil and partially hydrogenated oil
Vegetable oils are obtained from a variety of plants. Examples are sunflower, safflower, soya bean and corn. Unlike coconut or olive oil which can be obtained by simply pressing and separating oil, extracting vegetable oil can be more difficult. One of the most common commercial methods of extraction is to dissolve oil in a solvent (usually petroleum-derived hexane) which is both a quick and relatively inexpensive process that also achieves a high yield. Once the oil is dissolved, the solvent and any impurities are removed. These oils are then deodorised to remove odours, and bleached to remove pigmentation[89].

If vegetable oil is going to be made into margarine or shortening (sometimes called vegetable fat), it may undergo an additional step called hydrogenation which makes oil solid at room temperature. Hydrogenation involves mixing vegetable oils with a metal catalyst and heating at high temperatures. Hydrogen gas is then pumped through the hot oil in a high-pressure reactor. Partial hydrogenation leaves oil spreadable and increases shelf life but creates trans-fat[90]. At the end of the process some form of colouring is usually applied to both vegetable oil and margarine.

To suggest that this process doesn't sit well with me is an understatement. I'm truly baffled every time I think about it but, if you put the use of solvents aside, these oils can make you fat.

Why vegetable oil and partially hydrogenated oil can make you gain excess weight
1. Most vegetable oils are high in omega-6, and when consumed in excess these oils can cause too much inflammation in the body and encourage fat accumulation (see page 32).
2. Partially hydrogenated oil (which contains trans-fat) is like a double blow to weight loss attempts. Not only is it high in omega-6, being chemically altered, it's far removed from its natural state to the extent that the body doesn't recognise it as "real food". This can trigger a sequence of events that causes chronic food-induced inflammation resulting in "toxic fat".

When cooking, opt for non-hydrogenated olive or coconut oil which are both relatively low in omega-6 and provide other health benefits but avoid using these oils for high-temperature frying or baking to retain nutrient content and prevent formation of toxic compounds.

I've mentioned that "I try" to avoid vegetable oils as this is a tricky one that can go under the radar. Vegetable oils, particularly sunflower oil is often added to many foods that are considered to be healthy such as hummus, salad dressing, olives, granola and nut snack bars so many of us are unaware that we could be fuelling the problem by eating these. Vegetable oil can also be found in other foods including soup, sauces, mayonnaise, ice cream, popcorn as well as commercially baked food such as bread, pizza, pastries, pies, cakes and biscuits. Plus, if we go to a restaurant or buy a takeaway, we don't have a debate about what oil our food is being cooked in. As partially hydrogenated oil is less likely to spoil, it prolongs the shelf life of food made with it so some manufacturers use it as do many restaurants because these oils tend to last longer, are relatively stable at high temperatures and don't need to be changed as often as others when used for frying.

Some manufacturers have eliminated man-made trans-fats from their products but others still use them. When buying pastries and other baked foods that do not list ingredients, I would assume that the product does contain man-made trans-fats unless the manufacturer states otherwise.

Although research on the link between dietary saturated fats and heart disease has theories on both sides of the fence, guidelines encourage low consumption of saturated fats. While the debate rumbles on, all agree that good fats are an essential part of a balanced diet.

You need to eat fat to burn fat.
Stored fat cannot be burned without new dietary fat. Fat helps absorb key nutrients that can release fat stores and will help maintain good muscle health[91]. Good fats are more satiating than carbs which can also assist weight loss.

An overview of the good and not so good fats

The good unsaturated fats – monounsaturated and polyunsaturated:

Monounsaturated fat found in:
1. Coconuts and coconut oil
2. Olives and olive oil
3. Raw nuts and seeds
4. Avocados

Monounsaturated fats help increase your metabolism and reduce belly fat[92,93].

Polyunsaturated fat found in:
1. Oily fish such as salmon, mackerel, sardines and herring
2. Walnuts and pine nuts
3. Soya beans
4. Flax seeds

Some sources of polyunsaturated fats such as walnuts and soya beans also contain omega-6 which is a type of fat you generally want to reduce to avoid excessive food-induced inflammation. However, food sources such as those listed above, provide the body with other nutrients unlike some man-made foods such as partially hydrogenated oils and so are beneficial when consumed within guidelines.

The not so good saturated fats should be limited especially from foods such as:
1. Processed meat products, including some sausages
2. Savoury snacks including pastries and pies
3. Biscuits and cakes

The ugly

Small amounts of natural trans-fats can be found in foods including meat and dairy products but man-made trans-fat from partially hydrogenated oil should be avoided. If food contains partially hydrogenated oil, it will be listed under ingredients. Look out for **hydrogenated oil/fat** and **vegetable fat/shortening** (often used as an alternative name to vegetable oil and can also contain trans-fat). Trans-fats can make you fatter and give you a bigger belly than other foods with the same calories based on research at Wake Forest University School of Medicine.

According to Lawrence L. Rudel, PhD (professor of pathology and biochemistry and head of the Lipid Sciences Research Program, US), diets rich in trans-fat can lead to higher body weight even when the total dietary calories are controlled and cause a redistribution of fat tissue into the abdomen. In a study, researchers fed monkeys a Western-style diet where 35% of their diet was fat with half of the group receiving increased trans-fat, while others were fed unsaturated fats such as olive oil.

Over 6 years, monkeys fed a Western-style diet that contained trans-fat had a 7.2% increase in body weight, compared to a 1.8% increase in those that ate monounsaturated fats. All the extra weight went to the abdomen, and some other body fat was redistributed to the abdomen. Scans showed that the trans-fat group had dramatically more abdominal fat than the others. Both types of diets received the same calorie intake. Rudel and

Kavanagh explained. "We believed they couldn't get obese because we did not give them enough calories to get fat. We conclude that in equivalent diets, trans-fatty acid consumption increases weight gain[94]."

If you consume a lot of vegetable oils, takeaways, snacks and packaged foods, have excess belly fat and struggle to lose weight, this is likely to be the main cause due to excessive food-induced inflammation. Inflammation will disrupt your body's ability to burn fat and encourage fat storage. Fish oil supplements (high in omega-3) have been observed to reduce inflammation in the body in clinical trials[95]. Counteract food-induced inflammation with high quality fish or flax seed oil supplements.

Fat and hormones
Ironically, fat is the only macronutrient that doesn't directly stimulate the release of our main fat storing hormone, insulin. Although our body releases other fat storing hormones such as **acylation stimulating protein (ASP)** which is triggered by eating fat, most experts agree that ASP results in significantly lower levels of fat storage than insulin. However, it's worth remembering that the combination of carbs and fat in excess can result in the presence of 2 fat storing hormones acting as a catalyst to accumulate fat fast.

This is something to bear in mind when choosing treats and why too much consumption of snacks such as crisps, cakes, chocolate, ice cream, milkshake and even healthier options like dried fruit and nut mix and sweetened nut bars can inhibit weight loss despite reducing total calorie intake.

Fat trap fact 7
Man-made trans-fats and excess vegetable oils can cause weight gain and significant belly fat. Choose non-hydrogenated oils and counteract excessive inflammation with oils rich in omega-3.

Chapter 9

It's a mind game

Most goals are achieved in the mind before any action is taken, and weight loss is no different. Once we make the decision to change and are truly committed to the cause, it will no longer be a question of "if" I achieve my goal but "when". Holding onto a clear mental image of what you want and why will keep your target within your grasp. Your reason for change needs to be significant enough to push you over inevitable bumps in the road. Your drive for change can be whatever works for you but should be specific. If you want to have more energy, what will you do once you have more energy? If you want to be fitter, what is fit for you? Complete a 10k run, if so, by when? Or if you want your clothes to fit better, set a date. If you struggle with a strong enough reason why, remember, above all else, your health is paramount.

Being overweight and inactive can cause metabolic syndrome – a medical term for a combination of high blood pressure, diabetes and obesity. These common conditions that are interlinked can put you at greater risk of heart disease, stroke and other conditions affecting blood vessels[96].

Once we have a big enough reason why, we also need to be ready to tackle any mental obstacles that we often conjure up which can sabotage our efforts.

Have you ever found yourself staring into the fridge for no apparent reason, reached the bottom of a family-sized snack pack and you asked yourself, "Did I actually finish the whole lot," or simply notice if you turn to food as a source of comfort?

Emotional eating is very common and usually results in binge eating, but many of us don't even realise when we succumb to it until it's too late. Sometimes our attachment and reaction to food in certain emotional states can be so deep rooted that it becomes automatic and goes undetected. Many of us use food to suppress emotions such as stress, boredom, and loneliness[97]. Contrary to popular belief, many people who are "in shape" also suffer from binge eating episodes, so it really is a universal topic that should be tackled unashamedly.

It's all well and good to suggest that we should sort out whatever is causing us emotional distress in a bid to keep weight down. Although releasing ourselves from emotional baggage makes perfect sense to me and will certainly be of benefit, the reality is, life will always throw some emotional curve balls our way. So in addition to taking reasonable steps to accept and/or detach ourselves from our woes, we should also focus on damage limitation.

If we're honest, a lot of what we eat that causes the most damage happens alone, behind closed doors. So having an open and honest conversation with yourself can help identify and tackle emotional eating head on. Ask yourself the following questions:

1. What are my "trigger" foods/drinks which send me into a spiral of eating badly?
2. When am I most susceptible to these trigger foods?

I'll go first:

1. My trigger foods are cakes, crisps and sweets (yes, sweets. I used to eat way too many, and every once in a while I still get caught out so I keep these firmly on my list. To this day if I open a packet of sweets the chances are I will polish them off in record time or stop eating when I feel slightly nauseous – whichever comes first!).

2. I am more susceptible to these foods when I'm hungry, peeved off about something, it's simply in front of me, have run out of healthier snacks, become overconfident with my weight maintenance achievement – "I've got this sussed now, I can eat what I want," or simply when I allow myself to eat them too often and get a taste for them.

Based on your answers you can focus on steps to try and prevent emotional eating.

Tips to help prevent emotional eating

1. **Remove temptation** – avoid keeping trigger foods in the house and avoid shopping for food when you're in an emotional state.
2. **Eat a meal before going food shopping** as you are more likely to buy unhealthy snacks when you are hungry.
3. **Eat at set times during the day to avoid mindless snacking,** so no munching simply because you happen to pass the kitchen.
4. **Buy multipack individually wrapped snacks instead of one large family-sized bag.** Let's not kid ourselves; it's a lot easier to munch through one large pack than it is to open several small packs without feeling slightly guilty.
5. **Use stress management techniques** to help reduce stress and anxiety.
6. **If sleep deprivation is fuelling your binges,** use techniques suggested in chapter 5 to improve your sleep pattern and help balance hormones.
7. **Focus on feeding your cells nutritious foods daily** – trigger foods are usually unhealthy and initial cravings for unhealthy foods can also be a sign of nutrient deficiencies.
8. **Allow yourself one or two "treats" a week** so you have something to look forward to as a reward for eating well.
9. **Wait before you indulge** – emotional hunger comes on suddenly and usually needs to be satisfied instantly. Physical hunger can wait. Try and hold out for 15 minutes or so before giving in.
10. **Fill your spare time** with exercise, walks or a hobby to avoid eating out of boredom.

If you succumb to an eating frenzy try not to dwell on it. Draw a line under any setbacks and don't use it as an excuse to go the whole hog.

Fat trap fact 8
Be aware of emotional eating – pre-empt and focus on prevention.

Chapter 10

Realistic targets

It's all about results
One of the main reasons we abandon our efforts at weight loss is due to lack of results. Without consistent results we will become frustrated and are more likely to go back to eating what we ate before. The problem is, by the time we decide to lose weight, we want it gone yesterday. It goes without saying; weight gain that has taken months or even years to accumulate will take some time to lose.

Set realistic goals
Your overall weight loss target should be driven by how much weight you need to lose to be within your healthy weight category. If setting weekly targets, it is worth bearing in mind that losing more than 1–3 pounds a week is likely to result in losing proportionally more muscle mass than fat which, in the long-run, will make further weight loss and maintenance harder. We need to let go of the desire to find a quick fix. Targets should be realistic to sustain motivation and keep your metabolism fired up. Depending on how much weight you aim to lose, up to 3 pounds per week is a realistic target. If you focus on fat burn and eating well you can deliver significant visible results within weeks which can be achieved without becoming an obsessive bore that turns into a social hermit through fear of gorging on bad food.

The average adult has around 30 billion fat cells[98]. In general, when we gain weight gradually we increase the size of our fat cells. However, if weight gain is significant or sudden, **new fat cells can be created** to accommodate more fat storage[99]. Once we develop new fat cells we are stuck with them unless we have the willpower to shrink the cells (by losing weight) and maintain weight loss over a long period of time which can eventually induce cell death (apoptosis). The more fat cells we have the harder it is to lose weight as they are created for the purpose of storing fat – and are good at it! To avoid forming additional fat cells we need to monitor our weight on a regular basis as it's very easy to put on half a stone or more without even realising.

Standard weighing scales only give us one part of a weight loss story. If your overall weight goes down but body fat percentage increases, you can be lighter on the scales but proportionally fatter in shape which is generally not the desired look. If you want to be slim, healthy and look lean and toned – nothing wrong with that – it's important to try and keep on top of your body composition (fat, muscle and water percentage) along with waist and hip measurements to get the whole picture. Body composition scales/analysis can help identify muscle and fat percentage. Muscle weighs more than fat, as does bone, and any good exercise routine will aim to increase both muscle mass and bone density through weight bearing exercise. Pound for pound, fat occupies more space than muscle in the body. So if you increase muscle mass and bone density, you may increase your weight but shrink the size of your waist and become more toned. Burning fat and gaining muscle will result in losing inches.

Simply aiming to lose weight can result in muscle wastage which can leave you with a less desirable **"slim-fat"** look – when you are within your healthy weight but have high body fat percentage with relatively low muscle mass – and are likely to carry unwanted pounds around the belly. Increased muscle mass and fat burn while maintaining your weight would be beneficial.

Although stepping on the scales can be daunting, especially after an indulgent weekend, studies show that people who weigh themselves regularly lose more weight than those who don't[100]. Monitoring your weight will keep your goals in mind prompting you to act and avoid the classic head-in-the-sand syndrome of weight gain denial. We don't want this routine to become obsessive, agonising over every pound, given that your weight can fluctuate a few pounds within a day. Weekly (for standard scales) or monthly (body composition) weigh-ins should suffice while avoiding paranoia.

To achieve consistent and reliable readings when monitoring your weight, try to:

- Use the same weighing scales.
- Weigh yourself at the same time of day, on the same day of the week and in the same location of your home (as changes in flooring can alter your reading).

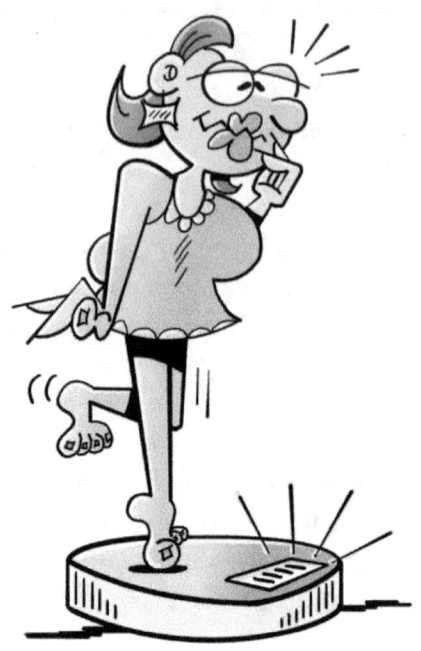

This might sound a bit OTT but it can make a difference.

Measurements can be taken:

- Waist – over bellybutton.
- Hips – over widest part.

Alternatively, have a set of clothes that are not elasticated at the waist which you can use to gauge potential weight loss based on how well your clothing fit you on a monthly basis to help monitor your progress.

Fat trap fact 9
Set realistic targets – monitor your weight weekly (for standard scales) or monthly (for body composition scales). Keep tabs on your body composition percentages and measurements to ensure you are losing fat not muscle.

Chapter 11

"Superfoods" and supplements

Some of us regularly scour the shelves of health food shops in a bid to find the next eagerly awaited superfood, hanging on the hope that it will assist in propelling our health and fitness kick. We don't need to purchase the latest "must have" weight loss aid sourced from around the world to achieve our goals. If you think about it, the absence of these superfoods we didn't know existed is not what makes us gain weight in the first place. Besides, there are many superfoods already at our beck and call, some a lot closer to home.

Water
Water contains minerals including calcium, magnesium and potassium – all for zero calories!

Simply drinking water can help you burn calories. The *Journal of Clinical Endocrinology & Metabolism* in 2003 observed that participants who drank 500ml of water temporarily boosted their metabolism, burning an additional 24 calories. Drinking 2 litres of water per day can result in burning nearly 100 calories[101].

In addition to this, water helps:
- Support daily detoxification, flushing out toxins.
- Maintains "normal" bowel function preventing constipation.
- Aids digestion, is essential to absorb water soluble nutrients and helps to remove excess water soluble nutrients from the body.
- Prevents cramps and sprains by keeping joints lubricated and muscles pliable – reducing the chance of injury.
- Thirst is often mistaken for hunger so staying hydrated can help prevent cravings.

Water helps every cell in our body function properly. Without it we would literally grind to a halt. Ok, so water is not food but the sentiment is the same – I think I'm on safe ground suggesting that water is a "superdrink" and many of us generally don't drink enough of it.

Remember to sip water throughout the day to allow absorption, and be aware of water intoxication (hyponatremia) which can be caused by over hydration. Although hyponatremia from consuming too much water is rare, it is important to be mindful of your daily intake and consume slowly during the course of the day.

If you drink tap water consider investing in a filter which can help remove potential unwanted substances.

Although there is no formal definition, it is generally accepted that superfoods are rich in nutrients and considered to be beneficial for health and wellbeing. Superfoods can assist with weight loss:

Avocado – packed with nearly 20 essential nutrients including vitamins E and B complex, avocados are the ultimate superfood and are a nutrient booster that contains monounsaturated fat which is more likely to be used as slow burning energy than stored as body fat.

Whole eggs contain 13 nutrients including vitamins D, B12 and A, and minerals such as iron and selenium. High in protein, eggs contain virtually no carbs and are low in calories. As the yolk contains the majority of its nutrients, organic, free-range whole eggs are preferred. Eggs were previously in the doghouse for containing cholesterol, however, several studies have questioned this link and there is currently no recommended limit on eggs as part of a varied diet[102,103].

Flax seeds – high in fibre and omega-3, and also provides iron, magnesium and calcium.

Quinoa – a seed which acts like a grain. Quinoa contains a balance of all amino acids making it a complete protein unlike most other vegetable sources of protein. It is also a good source of magnesium, B12 and high in fibre.

Cinnamon (celyon) – research suggests that cinnamon can help improve blood glucose levels and increase insulin sensitivity[104]. High in iron, magnesium and vitamin K, cinnamon is naturally sweet so is a good replacement for sugar.

Organic powdered super greens – rich in B vitamins and has a high protein to carbs ratio, can help curb cravings, support fat burn and promote a good night's sleep (if taken at least 3 hours before going to bed).

Seaweed – a good source of iodine, supports healthy function of thyroid glands which regulate metabolism, and is high in fibre assisting your body's normal detoxification process.

Mushrooms – the unsung heroes of superfoods. Not only are mushrooms low in energy, versatile and quick to cook, one serving can provide seven essential nutrients – riboflavin, niacin, pantothenic acid, biotin, copper, chromium and selenium.

Dark leafy greens and cruciferous vegetables are rich in many nutrients and low in energy. **Sprouts** including alfalfa, watercress and brussels sprouts can offer some of the highest levels of nutrition. Watercress, for example, has 17 nutrients, including potassium, fibre, protein, calcium, iron, thiamin, riboflavin, niacin, folate, zinc, and vitamins A, B6, B12, C, D, E, and K[105]. These vegetables should form part of our staple daily intake.

Supplements

There is definitely no shortage of supplements to choose from but we want to focus on ones that are not detrimental to your health – some options are:

Conjugated linoleic acid (CLA) – a group of compounds found in fatty acids, naturally present in dairy products and meat. Studies show significant reduction of body fat when CLA supplements are taken over a 12-week period (with majority of fat lost from the belly)[106,107].

Whey concentrate protein powder – a complete protein derived from milk containing all of the essential amino acids. Whey protein is one of the best sources of branched-chain amino acids (BCAAs) known to improve exercise performance and reduce muscle breakdown. Protein powder has been shown to stimulate rebuilding of muscle, when consumed soon after exercise (within about 30 minutes), increase calorie burn and suppress cravings. All protein powders are not equal; opt for organic grass fed, hormone free, cold pressed, whey protein concentrate (isolate goes through an additional step to remove remaining lactose and fat). Protein powder should be used as an addition to, but not a replacement for, whole foods so limit to 2–3 times per week. Consuming cow's milk in addition to your meals can cause weight gain – all milk from mammals is naturally designed to make infants grow. Ideally, mix protein powder with water or coconut milk or a mixture of milk and water.

Psyllium husk – derived from the plant plantango ovate (plantain), a source of soluble fibre, supports digestive health and normal bowel movement, assists detoxification by cleansing the system of waste, promotes good bacteria and reduces hunger by keeping you fuller for longer. Psyllium husk can make weight loss significantly easier and help flatten your belly. Add to smoothies, protein shakes or take before meals mixed with water – consume immediately. Drink at least 250ml of liquid with every teaspoon and consume sufficient water throughout the day. Taking psyllium husk without sufficient water can cause constipation.

Probiotics – supports immune function and aids digestion improving nutrient absorption. Studies show increased weight loss over a period of 12 weeks[108]. Just a heads up – there may be a period while good takes over bad which can result in loose stools.

Food based multivitamins – RDA / Recommended Daily Intake (RDI) are guidelines – the more active you are, the more nutrients your body requires. Micronutrients support multiple functions including thyroid health facilitating fat burn. Also ensure you are consuming sufficient vitamin D and magnesium. Vitamin D is used by every cell in the body, and low levels are often observed in people who are overweight. If you have dark skin, live where there is little sunshine and you generally cover your arms and legs, it's highly likely you are deficient in vitamin D; 1,000 IU of vitamin D3 daily would be beneficial particularly during the winter.

Fresh lemon juice aids digestion improving your body's ability to absorb nutrients, reduces hunger, stimulates the production of bile which can help the liver burn fat, and acts as a natural fat blocker reducing the amount of dietary fat absorbed by fat cells (due to pectin). Lemons also help flush the liver and kidneys of waste and toxins. All this from a humble lemon!

Green tea – increases your body's fat burn ability, can improve insulin sensitivity and binds to fat in the stomach preventing fat storage. Catechin, an antioxidant, found in green tea increases your metabolism by making it easier for your body to use excess body fat[109].

Fish oil/flax seed oil is rich in omega-3. Not only is fish oil a potent anti-inflammatory supplement, it can help reduce muscle protein breakdown and support muscle growth. Fish oil supplements are a great way to get some of the benefits of oily fish without potential pollutants that can accumulate in fatty fish. Opt for traceable and sustainable sources.

Chapter 12

One size doesn't fit all

Although a fully prescribed meal plan will leave less to interpretation, when you come off the plan, weight loss can be short-lived as it's easy to revert back to old habits causing weight to creep back on. It's important to make some daily food choices yourself in order to learn and build a healthy diet that works for you indefinitely. To some extent, a good weight loss programme should be modified to you as one size doesn't fit all.

Ideally, your weight loss programme should take into account the basics including your target weight and starting position, but also incorporate other areas within your control that extend beyond food. Changes should be moderate and sustainable with a view to improve your diet and lifestyle over a period of time. I'm always amazed by the number of people I speak to that go from no exercise at all to exercising 6 days a week and sometimes twice in a day – commendable, but will you maintain it? I think it's better to commit to exercise once or twice a week indefinitely than 6 times a week for a few weeks followed by months of exercise drought. Consider exercise as a necessity and remember to challenge yourself.

Depending on your current routine, a good quick start programme would be to:
1. **Alternate your breakfast**, especially if you eat cereal or toast daily (see recipe ideas).
2. **Incorporate a 5 a day salad** and bowl of mixed non-starchy vegetables daily.
3. **Avoid man-made trans-fat and limit vegetable oils** – supplement your diet with omega-3 oils.
4. **Try and restrict added and natural sugars** from food and drinks (excluding fresh fruit) to around 6 teaspoons a day.
5. **Workout at least once a week** (or more if you already do so).

Bodily functions such as fat storage and the release of hormones happen for a reason. If we didn't produce cortisol in times of stress we could keel over from shock, and, even if we did survive, we would constantly feel knackered without it. In the absence of insulin, blood sugars could rise to toxic levels. Hormones become an issue and cause weight gain if they are out of balance where the body produces too much or too little. Our focus therefore should be to try and bring balance – balance between nutrients, exercise and rest, work and play.

The human body is an amazing, intricate system wired for survival, and maintaining a healthy weight is critical to survival and already inbuilt. So how did our inbuilt weight balance mechanism become so skewed? Reduced nutrient content in food, over stimulation of taste buds from high energy, refined, rich foods that bypass our natural "stop eating" sensors, increased sugar and trans-fat intake along with pollutants and a sedentary stressful lifestyle have all contributed to a shift in our natural weight equilibrium. When foods are highly processed, refined and significantly altered from their natural state, they lack the nutrients to nourish our cells which have ramifications throughout the body. However, when you put the pieces of a weight loss puzzle together, you'll be surprised just how effective and fast weight loss can actually be. Even if you have more than your fair share of fat cells, are predisposed to storing fat, or can't remember the last time you were at your target weight, you can still regain control. Our bodies can be highly adaptable when we give it what it needs – it can reset.

If you take away only 3 points from reading this book, I hope it is the understanding that:

1. **Weight gain is a symptom and by-product of an impaired diet and lifestyle, both of which can be amended if we pull the right levers.**

2. **Eating fewer calories and exercising more may not lead to long-term weight loss or fat burn.**

3. **There is a science to fat burn**

Why conventional dieting often misses the mark.
Most conventional diets don't work in the long-term, but if you've ever tried them you probably know that already, and it's certainly not due to lack of trying. I often hear that weight loss is hard. I agree to an extent because if it were easy everyone would be at their desired weight but, if the tools and methods we use to lose weight are outdated and subpar for the task, it makes the job harder than it needs to be.

The concept of reducing calories to lose weight dates back to early 1900s before the hormones leptin and ghrelin were discovered, and before an understanding of how to burn fat were well established. In short, research has moved on. Simply restricting calories to lose weight is like trying to chop down a tree with an axe while a chainsaw lies idle beside you. You might get there eventually, but it would be a whole lot easier with the right tool as long as you know how to use it. Reduced calorie intake often results in both fat and muscle loss where the ratio of fat to muscle loss is dependent on how drastic calories are reduced, and the impact on nutrient intake. If your cells do not get sufficient nutrients, your metabolism can slow down significantly. Eating less food can result in higher levels of ghrelin (hunger hormone) and lower leptin (appetite suppressant hormone) which will work against you – no one likes the feeling of hunger and it's hard not to respond to it by stuffing your face. And even if you do have the willpower to restrict calories, a period of overeating is usually round the corner.

Leptin levels can fall drastically after just 7 days of significantly restricting calories making you feel ravenous! While leptin levels are low, your body's ability to burn fat dramatically decreases – your body is not aware of your desire to lose weight. All it knows is that you are eating less food and automatically wants to conserve energy and stock up. Some refer to this as **"starvation mode"**, an evolutionary survival mechanism we would be grateful for in times of famine, only some of us are yet to experience a famine. These reasons are fundamentally why conventional calorie-restricted diets often result in higher body fat percentage despite being lighter in weight.

Our focus should not actually be on weight loss but rather fat burn. To burn fat you need muscle, and muscle will not grow in the midst of food and nutrient scarcity. We actually want to focus on eating more – more mixed non-starchy, high-fibre vegetables, more healthy fats, plus enough quality protein for your body weight and activity level while restricting sugar and limiting vegetable oils. When we get this balance right you are likely to consume less energy automatically and develop more muscle mass.

No matter how hard you workout in the gym, a poor diet will keep your weight loss targets out of reach. The majority of fat burn comes down to the food we eat, the rest being exercise, genes, and other factors. Food impacts virtually everything from balancing hormones, energy levels and muscle growth to level of internal toxicity and quality of sleep.

Fat burn is more about balancing macronutrients to control fat storing hormones, feeding cells sufficient micronutrients from real foods, reducing excessive food-induced inflammation and preventing habitual binge eating than it is about restricting calories because the body does not use all calories in the same way.

The science of fat burn

As a friend quite rightly pointed out, fat burn is a science and sometimes science can be counter-intuitive or yield unexpected results. There's a formula to fat burn – the more you follow the formula, the faster you will see results.

Fat burn formula

Restrict sugar, refined carbs and high GL foods to reduce fat storing **insulin spikes.**

Short challenging exercise to release **glucagon** and bursts of adrenalin hormone.

Consume enough **protein** to help increase muscle mass and boost metabolism.

Maintain **low cortisol** levels using stress management techniques.

Support **high leptin** levels with appropriate calorie intake and regular quality sleep.

Restrict processed foods and focus on **feeding cells** a balance of nutrients.

Eliminate man-made, **inflammatory trans-fat** and up omega-3 intake to help release toxic fat.

Eat enough **good fats** to promote fat burn.

Reduce and help cleanse the body of **toxins.**

Have a positive mindset and pre-empt emotional eating.

Steps in pulling together your programme to support fat burn

1. **Make a note of your stats** including measurements and BMI. Use BMI chart to identify your healthy weight zone (in pounds on page 77 and kg page 78), and obtain your body composition using body analysis scales. BMI is a measure to help identify if you are overweight or obese and works for many individuals. However, it does not discriminate between fat and muscle, so if you have a high percentage of muscle mass (and few people who are overweight do), it will not work for you as muscle weighs more than fat. In this case, you can focus on measurements and body composition readings.
2. **In addition to exercise, focus on 2 weight loss inhibitors** listed on page 75. Work through the summary of 10 weight loss inhibitors and select 2 areas of focus (plus exercise) that are pertinent to you based on possible signs, and revisit relevant chapters.
3. **Choose one Food Plan approach** to help control fat storing hormone, insulin. Either:
   - Monitor carbs daily by grams while opting for low glycemic load foods, or
   - Two non-consecutive fat burn low-carb days with one treat day per week.

   Both plans should incorporate sufficient calorie and protein intake.
4. **Plan your week**. Using exercise suggestions, food plans, top tips and recipe ideas, pull together a weekly programme that you can commit to. The aim is to get an idea of what a **good day** and **good week** looks like for you while incorporating nutrient boosters such as 5 a day salads, vegetable juice and superfoods without getting bogged down with the minutiae on a day to day basis. Once you have an idea of a good day/week, rotate food choices and repeat.
5. **Follow your plan wholeheartedly**. Keep your weekly programme close to hand and follow for 4 weeks before making any changes. Let go of any preconceived ideas, be positive and focus on the prize!

Top 10 Tips for fat burn

1. **To prevent appetite suppressing leptin levels from falling** avoid reducing calories drastically and opt for moderate reduction – up to 20% lower than your normal calorie intake. Alternatively, focus your efforts on 2–3 non-consecutive, low-carb, fat burn days per week followed by one day where you allow yourself foods you want so your body knows that food is not in short supply and maintains normal fat burn activity – keeping your hormones balanced.

2. **Protein.** Many studies show that increasing protein intake can lead to automatic weight loss and one study reported a decrease of 441 calories (19% less) when subjects increased protein intake from 15% to 30% of calories [110,111,112,113]. Based on a 2000-calorie diet, eating more protein can result in 380 fewer calories a day without even trying!

3. **Restrict fruit juices.** One medium glass of orange juice can include up to 5 oranges which would be equal to around 75 grams of sugar (83% of GDA [90g]). It's very easy to go over the recommended maximum sugar intake when drinking fruit juice which can contribute to belly fat. Opt to eat or blend fruit instead, maximising fibre intake. One cup of **mixed vegetable juice** on the other hand is a great way to up nutrient intake and detox your taste buds.

4. **Breakfast doesn't have to come out of a box.** People are often at a loss when choosing what to eat for breakfast and I try not to sound sarcastic when I simply suggest… food. The habit of eating cereal for breakfast started to take a hold in the early 1900s, but before cereal we simply ate food and many cultures still do[114,115]. Most cereals are effectively processed starchy carbs (either processed wheat or rice) and are likely to make you start the day burning and wanting more sugar. Consider rotating your breakfast choices and start your day with nutrient dense foods such as superfoods or vegetable juices (alternatively, opt for cereals with no added sugar and preferably little or no dried fruit).

5. **Most wheat based foods breed belly fat.** Wheat and wheat based foods such as pasta, breads, bagels, cereals, pretzels, breadsticks, crackers and muffins often contain a starch (carb) called amylopectin-A and gluten. Amylopectin-A raises blood sugar more than other carbs, increasing insulin and stimulating cravings, while gluten can cause

inflammation in the body. A combination of amylopectin-A and gluten can result in belly fat which some refer to as **"wheat belly"**. Try and think of wheat as a treat, not a daily staple. Standard potatoes also contain high levels of amylopectin-A and should be restricted.

6. **Short on time?** Prepare as much food as possible in batches while minimising nutrient loss. It takes about the same amount of time to grill 4 portions of chicken as it does to grill 1, and as meat and poultry retain fat soluble vitamins relatively well you can freeze uneaten portions and defrost during the course of the week. Prepare 2–3 portions of 5 a day salad (without dressing) and keep refrigerated. Frozen vegetables are also a great way to have veg on tap.

7. **Timing of your meals matter.** If you are overweight the chances are you have high insulin levels throughout the day and are therefore more inclined to store fat. If you eat a high energy meal including starchy carbs late at night, with little activity before or after, you are likely to store the majority of your meal as fat given that you are predisposed to store fat and because our metabolism naturally slows down in the evening in preparation for sleep. If you skip breakfast and don't eat much throughout the day your metabolism will remain low and you are more likely to have cravings in the evening which can encourage binge eating. Work towards eating your main starchy meals during the day around lunch time when your metabolism is usually near its peak and try to keep evening meals light, consuming mainly lean protein and non-starchy veg.

8. **Alcohol counts too.** A pint of beer provides the same calories as a packet of crisps, and a standard bottle of alcopop gives you the same energy as three teacakes. If you drink alcohol keep an eye on how much alcohol you consume as unused energy can quickly add up[116]. It is best considered a treat so consume a maximum of 2 drinks per week.

9. **One for the ladies.** Premenstrual Syndrome (PMS) symptoms are not only linked to throwing a wobbly every now and then. There are up to 150 known symptoms which can occur within 2 weeks of your menstrual period and include; fatigue, cravings, increased hunger and weight gain of anything up to 10 pounds due to changes in hormone levels which can result in water retention[117,118]. Weight gain due to PMS is usually short-lived but if you succumb to cravings and binge eat, you may gain fat. Be aware of your menstrual cycle and use

73

suggestions in chapter 9 to prevent unhealthy food choices. Avoid scheduling a fat burn day within 3 days of the start of your period when your appetite generally ramps up.

10. **Portion size matters,** especially for "insulin spiking" starchy carbs including grains which generally provide limited nutritional value when compared to non-starchy vegetables. If you're out and about or simply don't have the time or inclination to work out grams for each food group, use your hand to measure portions:

- **Unlimited**: Mixed non-starchy vegetables (including leafy greens).
- **Fist size**: Starch (e.g. rice, yam or pasta)/fruit.
- **Palm** (size and thickness): Meat/poultry/fish*.
- **Thumb**: Cheese.

Aim to fill at least half of your plate with mixed non-starchy vegetables for lunch and dinner.

* Fish – up to twice the size and thickness of your palm.

Weight loss inhibitor	Possible signs that indicate weight loss inhibitor	Chapter
Insufficient protein	Food cravings/hunger pangs Frequent colds and infections Low muscle tone/muscle soreness and cramps Weak/thinning hair Irregular periods/PMS due to hormone imbalance	2
Insufficient micronutrient intake	Poor skin/hair condition Frequent colds/infections/run-down symptoms White spots/brown bands on nails Excessive hunger/binge eating Significantly overweight	3
Not enough or too much exercise	Sleep problems/restlessness Lack of clarity Stress/depression Little or no muscle tone Frequent colds/infections	4
Not enough quality sleep	Increased appetite Not feeling rested upon waking/you fall asleep immediately at bed time/insomnia Abdominal fat Fatigued/dark cycles under eyes Poor concentration/poor memory/irritability	5
High levels of stress	Sleep problems/insomnia Food cravings Irritability/mood swings "Brain fog"/difficulty concentrating/poor memory Abdominal fat	5
Toxin Overload	Skin problems such as acne and eczema/poor skin quality Body odour, bad breath "Brain fog"/cognitive problems/headaches/sleep problems Fluid retention particularly around abdomen, ankles and feet (edema) Yellowish skin/eyes (symptom of jaundice)	6

Insulin resistance/red-uced insulin sensitivity	Significantly overweight/inability to lose weight/you're in the obese category of BMI Abdominal obesity/belly fat Excessive hunger/food cravings You regularly eat desserts/chocolate Your carbs are mainly from starchy veg, bread, potatoes, pasta and rice	7
Insufficient healthy fats/too many bad fats	Abdominal obesity/belly fat You regularly eat cakes, biscuits, crisps takeaways, fast foods, pastries or pies Mood swings (due to lack of serotonin)/"brain fog"/poor memory Dry/flaky skin (due to poor vitamin absorption and oil production) Irregular periods/PMS due to hormone imbalance	8
Emotional eating	You're not hungry enough to eat a portion of fruit but can devour a cake Binge eating followed by guilt Your cravings feel intense and out of control You go to great lengths to get the food you want like taking a detour You can mindlessly eat family size snacks in one sitting	9
Unrealistic targets	Your weight yo-yos up and down You find the process of weight loss way too hard You expect to lose more than 3 pounds per week When you fall off the wagon, you really fall off!	10

BMI Checker (weight in pounds)

Find your height along the top or bottom of grid then find your nearest weight in the same vertical column within the grid. Look for BMI in horizontal row level with your weight along the borders.

Height in Feet & inches

4' 11" 5' 0" 5' 1" 5' 2" 5' 3" 5' 4" 5' 5" 5' 6" 5' 7" 5' 8" 5' 9" 5' 10" 5' 11" 6' 0" 6' 1" 6' 2"

Height in inches

BMI	59	60	61	62	63	64	65	66	67	68	69	70	71	72	73	74	BMI
19	94	97	100	104	107	110	114	118	121	125	128	132	136	140	144	148	19
20	99	102	106	109	113	116	120	124	127	131	135	139	143	147	151	155	20
21	104	107	111	115	118	122	126	130	134	138	142	146	150	154	159	163	21
22	109	112	116	120	124	128	132	136	140	144	149	153	157	162	166	171	22
23	114	118	122	126	130	134	138	142	146	151	155	160	165	169	174	179	23
24	119	123	127	131	135	140	144	148	153	158	162	167	172	177	182	186	24
25	124	128	132	136	141	145	150	155	159	164	169	174	179	184	189	194	25
26	128	133	137	142	146	151	156	161	166	171	176	181	186	191	197	202	26
27	133	138	143	147	152	157	162	167	172	177	182	188	193	199	204	210	27
28	138	143	148	153	158	163	168	173	178	184	189	195	200	206	212	218	28
29	143	148	153	158	163	169	174	179	185	190	196	202	208	213	219	225	29
30	148	153	158	164	169	174	180	186	191	197	203	209	215	221	227	233	30
31	153	158	164	169	175	180	186	192	198	203	209	216	222	228	235	241	31
32	158	163	169	175	180	186	192	198	204	210	216	222	229	235	242	249	32
33	163	168	174	180	186	192	198	204	211	216	223	229	236	242	250	256	33
34	168	174	180	186	191	197	204	210	217	223	230	236	243	250	257	264	34
35	173	179	185	191	197	204	210	216	223	230	236	243	250	258	265	272	35
36	178	184	190	196	203	209	216	223	230	236	243	250	257	265	272	280	36
37	183	189	195	202	208	215	222	229	236	243	250	257	265	272	280	287	37
38	188	194	201	207	214	221	228	235	242	249	257	264	272	279	288	295	38
39	193	199	206	213	220	227	234	241	249	256	263	271	279	287	295	303	39
40	198	204	211	218	225	232	240	247	255	262	270	278	286	294	302	311	40
41	203	209	217	224	231	238	246	253	261	269	277	285	293	302	310	319	41
42	208	215	222	229	237	244	252	260	268	276	284	292	301	309	318	326	42
43	212	220	227	235	242	250	258	266	274	282	291	299	308	316	325	334	43
44	217	225	232	240	248	256	264	272	280	289	297	306	315	324	333	342	44
45	222	230	238	246	254	262	270	278	287	295	304	313	322	331	340	350	45
46	227	235	243	251	259	267	276	284	293	302	311	320	329	338	348	358	46
47	232	240	248	256	265	273	282	291	299	308	318	327	338	346	355	365	47
48	237	245	254	262	270	279	288	297	306	315	324	334	343	353	363	373	48
49	242	250	259	267	278	285	294	303	312	322	331	341	351	361	371	381	49
50	247	255	264	273	282	291	300	309	319	328	338	348	358	368	378	389	50
51	252	261	269	278	287	296	306	315	325	335	345	355	365	375	386	396	51
52	257	266	275	284	293	302	312	322	331	341	351	362	372	383	393	404	52
53	262	271	280	289	299	308	318	328	338	348	358	369	379	390	401	412	53
54	267	276	285	295	304	314	324	334	344	354	365	376	386	397	408	420	54
55	272	281	290	300	310	320	330	340	351	361	372	383	393	404	416	428	55

150 152 155 157 160 163 165 168 170 173 175 178 180 183 185 188

Height in Centimetres

☐ 19–24 Healthy   ▨ 25–29 Overweight   ▩ 30+ Obese

BMI Checker (weight in Kg)

Find your height along the top or bottom of grid then find your nearest weight in the same vertical column within the grid. Look for BMI in horizontal row level with your weight along the borders.

Height in Feet & inches

| 4'11" | 5'0" | 5'1" | 5'2" | 5'3" | 5'4" | 5'5" | 5'6" | 5'7" | 5'8" | 5'9" | 5'10" | 5'11" | 6'0" | 6'1" | 6'2" |

Height in inches

BMI	59	60	61	62	63	64	65	66	67	68	69	70	71	72	73	74	BMI
19	43	44	45	47	49	50	52	54	55	57	58	60	62	64	65	67	19
20	45	46	48	49	51	53	54	56	58	59	61	63	65	67	68	70	20
21	47	49	50	52	54	55	57	59	61	63	64	66	68	70	72	74	21
22	49	51	53	54	56	58	60	62	64	65	68	69	71	73	75	78	22
23	52	54	55	57	59	61	63	64	66	68	70	73	75	77	79	81	23
24	54	56	58	59	61	64	65	67	69	72	73	76	78	80	83	84	24
25	56	58	60	62	64	66	68	70	72	74	77	79	81	83	86	88	25
26	58	60	62	64	66	68	71	73	75	78	80	82	84	87	89	92	26
27	60	63	65	67	69	71	73	76	78	80	83	85	88	90	93	95	27
28	63	65	67	69	72	74	76	78	81	83	86	88	91	93	96	99	28
29	65	67	69	72	74	77	79	81	84	86	89	92	94	97	99	102	29
30	67	69	72	74	77	79	82	84	87	89	92	95	98	100	103	106	30
31	69	72	74	77	79	82	84	87	90	92	95	98	101	103	107	109	31
32	72	74	77	79	82	84	87	90	93	95	98	101	104	107	110	113	32
33	74	76	79	82	84	87	90	93	96	98	101	104	107	110	113	116	33
34	76	79	82	84	87	89	93	95	98	101	104	107	110	113	117	120	34
35	78	81	84	87	89	93	95	98	101	104	107	110	113	117	120	123	35
36	81	83	86	89	92	95	98	101	104	107	110	113	117	120	123	127	36
37	83	86	88	92	94	98	101	104	107	110	113	117	120	123	127	130	37
38	85	88	91	94	97	100	103	107	110	113	117	120	123	127	131	134	38
39	88	90	93	97	100	103	106	109	113	116	119	123	127	130	134	137	39
40	90	93	96	99	102	105	109	112	116	119	122	126	130	133	137	141	40
41	92	95	98	102	105	108	112	115	118	122	126	129	133	137	141	145	41
42	94	98	101	104	108	111	114	118	122	125	129	132	137	140	144	148	42
43	96	100	103	107	110	113	117	121	124	128	132	136	140	143	147	151	43
44	98	102	105	109	112	116	120	123	127	131	135	139	143	147	151	155	44
45	101	104	108	112	115	119	122	126	130	134	138	142	146	150	154	159	45
46	103	107	110	114	117	121	125	129	133	137	141	145	149	153	158	162	46
47	105	109	112	116	120	124	128	132	136	140	144	148	153	157	161	166	47
48	108	111	115	119	122	127	131	135	139	143	147	151	156	160	165	169	48
49	110	113	117	121	126	129	133	137	142	146	150	155	159	164	168	173	49
50	112	116	120	124	128	132	136	140	145	149	153	158	162	167	171	176	50
51	114	118	122	126	130	134	139	143	147	152	156	161	166	170	175	180	51
52	117	121	125	129	133	137	142	146	150	155	159	164	169	174	178	183	52
53	119	123	127	131	136	140	144	149	153	158	162	167	172	177	182	187	53
54	121	125	129	134	138	142	147	151	156	161	166	171	175	180	185	191	54
55	123	127	132	136	140	145	150	154	159	164	169	174	178	183	189	194	55

| 150 | 152 | 155 | 157 | 160 | 163 | 165 | 168 | 170 | 173 | 175 | 178 | 180 | 183 | 185 | 188 |

Height in Centimetres

19–24 Healthy   25–29 Overweight   30+ Obese

Age-adjusted body fat percentage[119]

If you have body composition scales, these tables can be used to interpret body fat percentage result.

Women

Age	Underweight	Healthy Range	Overweight	Obese
20–39 yrs	Under 21%	21–33%	33–39%	Over 39%
40–59 yrs	Under 23%	23–34%	34–40%	Over 40%
60–79 yrs	Under 24%	24–36%	36–42%	Over 42%

Men

Age	Underweight	Healthy Range	Overweight	Obese
20–39 yrs	Under 8%	8–20%	20–25%	Over 25%
40–59 yrs	Under 11%	11–22%	22–28%	Over 28%
60–79 yrs	Under 13%	13–25%	25–30%	Over 30%

Source: NIH/WHO guidelines for BMI
Source: Gallagher et al., American Journal of Clinical Nutrition, Vol. 72, Sept. 2000

Skeletal muscle percentages[120]

If you have body composition scales, this table can be used to interpret skeletal muscle percentage result.

Gender	Age	Low (-)	Normal (0)	High (+)	Very high (++)
Female	**18–39**	< 24.3	24.3–30.3	30.4–35.3	≥ 35.4
	40–59	< 24.1	24.1–30.1	30.2–35.1	≥ 35.2
	60–80	< 23.9	23.9–29.9	30.0–34.9	≥ 35.0
Male	**18–39**	< 33.3	33.3–39.3	39.4–44.0	≥ 44.1
	40–59	< 33.1	33.1–39.1	39.2–43.8	≥ 43.9
	60–80	< 32.9	32.9–38.9	39.0–43.6	≥ 43.7

Source: Omron Healthcare

Suggested average calorie intake[121]

Gender	Age	Sedentary	Moderately Active	Active	Very Active
Female	19–30	1800–2000	2000–2200	2400	2600+
	31–50	1800	2000	2200	2400+
	51+	1600	1800	2000–2200	2400+
Male	19–30	2400–2600	2600–2800	3000	3200+
	31–50	2200–2400	2400–2600	2800–3000	3400+
	51+	2000–2200	2200–2400	2400–2800	3000+

- **Sedentary:** Never or rarely include physical activity in your day.
- **Moderately active:** Include light or moderate activity two to three times a week.
- **Active:** At least 30 minutes of moderate activity most days or 20 minutes of vigorous activity at least three days a week.
- **Very active:** Include large amounts of moderate or vigorous activity in your day.

Suggested minimum protein intake guidelines vary but the following is generally accepted: 0.8 grams per kg of body weight for sedentary people going up to 1.4 or 1.8 grams if very active (or approximately 0.36 grams per pound going up to 0.82 grams if very active). Alternatively, work towards estimates below to support an effective fat burn programme.

Estimated protein intake in grams based on suggested calorie intake

Gender	Age	Sedentary	Moderately Active	Active	Very Active
Female	19–30	135–150	150–165	180	195+
	31–50	135	150	165	180+
	51+	120	135	150–165	180+
Male	19–30	180–195	195–210	225	240+
	31–50	165–180	180–195	210–225	255+
	51+	150–165	165–180	180–210	225+

Chapter 13

Cruise control

Weight maintenance

I'd love to say once you hit your target healthy weight it will be plain sailing, but that obviously isn't the case as it's easy to fall back into old habits, particularly if the process of losing fat was very restrictive. It becomes hard to find the middle ground between all and nothing.

There may be periods when you have less control of what is put on your plate – birthdays, christenings, weddings, holidays can all come at once and throw us off track – so from time to time you can expect to loosen your belt – literally! There are also times when you may have to pass on eating cake or take the smallest of slices to keep the balance.

The idea is if you focus on feeding your cells and fat burn is controlled, your metabolism should remain healthy. So even if you take a hiatus you are less likely to put weight back on rapidly. Eventually you will find what some call your **"feel-good weight"** at which you feel comfortable within yourself allowing for a middle ground so you can enjoy food and socialising with food on special occasions. This will come with trial and error and as long as you are within your healthy weight range it's not a bad place to be.

Tips for weight maintenance:

1. **Continue to monitor your stats regularly** and decide on a "cut-off" weight, around 7 pounds heavier than your target weight. If you hit your cut-off weight go back on your programme. The intention is to try and avoid hitting your cut-off weight.
2. **Use changes in your body as an indicator** of how clean and balanced your diet and lifestyle is. Consider changes to your skin and hair, whiteness of your eyes, quality of sleep, your general mood, how regular your bowel movements are and so on.

3. **Reward yourself occasionally** as deprivation often leads to temptation, and when you have a treat or snack take time to savour and appreciate it.
4. **Allow yourself to determine your food portion sizes** as opposed to what restaurants or what other people give you. Opt to share meals or take away uneaten/leftover food if need be.
5. **Focus on 1 fat burn day a week to help stay on track,** return to moderate protein consumption if you increased intake to 30% of calories unless you go back on your programme. Keep an eye on your nutrient intake from foods but give yourself some flexibility to find a new "normal" that fits you.

I've accepted that my childhood love for cakes, crisps and even sweets will, to an extent, forever exist, but now I also enjoy healthier foods and have more control over cravings. Although I have been within my healthy weight category since early adulthood, it is only in recent years I can finally say I have better control of my weight which doesn't actually come from achieving a washboard stomach or simply reaching and even maintaining your target weight, but from a sense of letting go of the fear of gaining weight.

As corny as it might sound, the best part of this process will be when you embed the main principles of fat burn into your lifestyle and stop worrying that the old you will return even when there are bumps in the road. When food is no longer your main topic of discussion, or a constant feature in your thoughts, but a means to sustain health and derive enjoyment, it is then that you can truly enjoy the freedom of being released from the fat trap.

Chapter 14

Programme ideas

Weight (weekly), BMI and body composition percentages (monthly)				
Your stats	**Week 1**	**Week 2**	**Week 3**	**Target**
Weight				
Muscle %				
Body Fat %				
Water %				
Waist (W)				
Hip (H)				
W / H Ratio				
BMI				
	Week 4	**Week 5**	**Week 6**	**Target**
Weight				
Muscle %				
Body Fat %				
Water %				
Waist (W)				
Hip (H)				
W / H Ratio				
BMI				
	Week 7	**Week 8**	**Week 9**	**Target**
Weight				
Muscle %				
Body Fat %				
Water %				
Waist (W)				
Hip (H)				
W / H Ratio				
BMI				

	Week 10	Week 11	Week 12	Target
Weight				
Muscle %				
Body Fat %				
Water %				
Waist (W)				
Hip (H)				
W / H Ratio				
BMI				
	Week 13	Week 14	Week 15	Target
Weight				
Muscle %				
Body Fat %				
Water %				
Waist (W)				
Hip (H)				
W / H Ratio				
BMI				
	Week 16	Week 17	Week 18	Target
Weight				
Muscle %				
Body Fat %				
Water %				
Waist (W)				
Hip (H)				
W / H Ratio				
BMI				
	Week 19	Week 20	Week 21	Target
Weight				
Muscle %				
Body Fat %				
Water %				
Waist (W)				
Hip (H)				
W / H Ratio				
BMI				

Food Plan Option 1. Monitor carbs daily. Maintain sufficient calorie, protein and fibre intake.

Food			Mon	Tue	Wed	Thu	Fri	Sat	Sun
Carbs	Grams		150–200	150–200	150–200	150–200	150–200	150–200	150–200
Breakfast	Options	1	Coconut yoghurt & strawberries	Breakfast salad	Coconut yoghurt & strawberries	Breakfast salad	Coconut yoghurt & strawberries	Breakfast salad	Coconut yoghurt & strawberries
		2	Porridge & mixed seeds topping	Porridge & mixed seeds topping	Porridge & mixed seeds topping	Porridge & mixed seeds topping	Porridge & mixed seeds topping	Porridge & mixed seeds topping	Porridge & mixed seeds topping
		3	2 eggs & avocado	2 eggs & avocado	2 eggs & avocado	2 eggs & avocado	2 eggs & avocado	2 eggs & avocado	2 eggs & avocado
		4	Breakfast salad	2 eggs & veg	Breakfast salad	2 eggs & veg	Breakfast salad	2 eggs & veg	Breakfast salad
		5	Creamy green juice	Protein shake	Creamy green juice	Protein shake	Creamy green juice	Protein shake	Creamy green juice
Lunch	Options	1	Usual food & non-starchy veg	Usual food & non-starchy veg	Usual food & non-starchy veg	Usual food & non-starchy veg	Usual food & non-starchy veg	Usual food & non-starchy veg	Usual food & non-starchy veg
		2	Poultry / meat / fish / pulses & non-starchy veg / salad	Poultry / meat / fish / pulses & non-starchy veg / salad	Poultry / meat / fish / pulses & non-starchy veg / salad	Poultry / meat / fish / pulses & non-starchy veg / salad	Poultry / meat / fish / pulses & non-starchy veg / salad	Poultry / meat / fish / pulses & non-starchy veg / salad	Poultry / meat / fish / pulses & non-starchy veg / salad
Dinner	Options	1	Usual food & 5 a day salad	Usual food & 5 a day salad	Usual food & 5 a day salad	Usual food & 5 a day salad	Usual food & 5 a day salad	Usual food & 5 a day salad	Usual food & 5 a day salad
		2	Poultry / meat / fish & veg / salad	Poultry / meat / fish & veg / salad	Poultry / meat / fish & veg / salad	Poultry / meat / fish & veg / salad	Poultry / meat / fish & veg / salad	Poultry / meat / fish & veg / salad	Poultry / meat / fish & veg / salad
Snacks	Options	1	1–2 portions of fruit	1–2 portions of fruit	1–2 portions of fruit	1–2 portions of fruit	1–2 portions of fruit	1–2 portions of fruit	1–2 portions of fruit
		2	Sugar snap peas	Green beans & 1 tbl homemade pesto	Sugar snap peas	Green beans & 1 tbl homemade pesto	Sugar snap peas	Green beans & 1 tbl homemade pesto	Sugar snap peas
		3	Cucumber & cottage cheese	Cucumber & cottage cheese	Cucumber & cottage cheese	Cucumber & cottage cheese	Cucumber & cottage cheese	Cucumber & cottage cheese	Cucumber & cottage cheese
		4	5 olives	10 raw cashews	5 olives	10 raw almonds	5 olives	10 raw walnuts	5 olives
		5	Half avocado	Half avocado	Half avocado	Half avocado	Half avocado	Half avocado	Half avocado

Portions if using your hand – Protein: size and thickness of palm. **Starchy carbs/fruit:** size of your fist. **Non starchy veg:** unlimited. **Cheese:** size of thumb

Red meat and oily fish – Red meat: no more than 70g per day. **Oily fish** (140g per portion): men up to 4 portions per week, women up to 2 portions per week.

Food Plan Option 2. Two non-consecutive, fat burn, low-carb/low GL days maintaining sufficient calorie, protein and fibre intake.

			Mon	Tue	Wed	Thu	Fri	Sat	Sun
			Maintain	Fat Burn	Maintain	Fat Burn	Maintain	Maintain	Treat
Carbs	Grams								
	Options	1	150–200	60–100	150–200	60–100	150–200	150–200	
		2	100–150	50–60	100–150	50–60	100–150	100–150	
Food	Breakfast								
	Options	1	Coconut yoghurt & strawberries	Breakfast salad	Coconut yoghurt & strawberries	Breakfast salad	Coconut yoghurt & strawberries	Breakfast salad	Coconut yoghurt & strawberries
		2	Porridge & mixed seeds topping	Creamy mushrooms & veg	Porridge & mixed seeds topping	Creamy mushrooms & veg	Porridge & mixed seeds topping	Porridge & mixed seeds topping	Porridge & mixed seeds topping
		3	2 eggs & veg	Creamy green juice	2 eggs & veg	Creamy green juice	2 eggs & veg	Creamy green juice	2 eggs & veg
		4	Breakfast salad	2 eggs & avocado	Breakfast salad	2 eggs & avocado	Breakfast salad	2 eggs & avocado	Breakfast salad
		5	Usual food	Protein shake	Usual food	Protein shake	Usual food	Usual food	Usual food
	Lunch								
	Options	1	Usual food & 5 a day salad	Soup / poultry / meat / fish & non-starchy veg / salad	Usual food & 5 a day salad	Soup / poultry / meat / fish & non-starchy veg / salad	Usual food & 5 a day salad	Usual food & 5 a day salad	Usual food & 5 a day salad
	Dinner								
	Options	1	Poultry / meat / fish / pulses & mixed non-starchy veg	Poultry / meat / fish & 1–2 cups of broccoli	Poultry / meat / fish / pulses & mixed non-starchy veg	Poultry / meat / fish & 1–2 cups of broccoli	Poultry / meat / fish / pulses & mixed non-starchy veg	**Treat meal**	**Treat meal**
	Snacks								
	Options	1	1–2 portions of fruit	Green beans & 1 tbl homemade pesto	1–2 portions of fruit	Green beans & 1 tbl homemade pesto	1–2 portions of fruit	1–2 portions of fruit	1–2 portions of fruit
		2	Sugar snap peas	Strawberries	Sugar snap peas	Strawberries	Sugar snap peas	Sugar snap peas	Sugar snap peas
		3	Cucumber & cottage cheese	Coconut yoghurt	Cucumber & cottage cheese	Coconut yoghurt	Cucumber & cottage cheese	Cucumber & cottage cheese	Cucumber & cottage cheese
		4	5 olives	10 raw cashews	5 olives	10 raw almonds	5 olives	10 raw walnuts	5 olives
		5	Half avocado	Half avocado	Half avocado	Half avocado	Half avocado	Half avocado	**1 Treat**

Portions if using your hand – Protein: size and thickness of palm. **Starchy carbs/fruit:** size of your fist. **Non starchy veg:** unlimited. **Cheese:** size of thumb.
Red meat and oily fish – Red meat: no more than 70g per day. **Oily fish** (140g per portion): men up to 4 portions per week, women up to 2 portions per week.

86

Food list ideas with estimated protein, carbs and calories. Aim to consume at least 30g of fibre per day plus your carb (page 48) and protein (page 80) intake.

Food List	Protein	Carbs	Fibre	Cal	Food List	Protein	Carbs	Fibre	Cal
	g	g	g			g	g	g	
Poultry/meat/fish/egg					**Non-starchy veg**				
Salmon 1 fillet (155g)	42	-	-	285	Mixed leaf salad 1 cup	1	2	1	10
Beef tenderloin (85g)	20	-	-	275	Kale 1 cup	1	1	1	8
Sardines 1 can (120g)	21	-	-	196	White mushroom 1 cup	2	2	1	15
Chicken breast (86g)	27	-	-	142	Cauliflower 1 cup	2	5	2	27
Lamb chop (85g)	24	-	-	261	Broccoli 1 cup	3	6	2	31
Mackerel fillet (88g)	21	-	-	231	Red sweet pepper	1	7	3	37
Chicken thigh with skin (137g)	32	-	-	318	Tomato medium	1	5	2	22
Tempeh (100g)	20	8	-	195	Okra (cooked) 8 pods	2	4	2	19
1 egg (medium)	6	0	-	65	Beets 1 cup	2	13	4	58
Whey protein concentrate (25g)	21	2	-	107	Carrots chopped 1 cup	1	12	4	52
					Celery 1 medium stalk	0	1	1	6
Starch					Green beans (55g)	1	4	2	17
Sweet potato cubes 1 cup (baked)	3	41	3	176	Onion (medium)	1	10	2	44
Yam cubes 1 cup (boiled)	2	37	5	158	Edamame 1 cup	17	15	8	189
Plantain 1 medium	2	68	5	253	10 sugar snap peas	1	3	1	14
Brown basmati rice (cooked) 1 cup	5	45	4	216	Soup (veg) 1 cup	4	12	2	98
White basmati rice (cooked) 1 cup	6	40	1	190					
Quinoa (cooked) 1 cup	8	39	5	222	**Dairy and non-dairy milk**				
Buckwheat groats (cooked) 1 cup	6	34	5	155	Cottage cheese (100g)	14	4	-	90
Egg noodles (cooked) 1 cup	7	40	2	221	Ricotta cheese (100g)	11	3	-	174
Oats dry half a cup	5	27	4	150	Greek yoghurt 170g pot	15	6	-	163
Sourdough bread 1 slice	2	13	1	68	Cow's whole milk 1/2 cup	4	6	-	73
					Coconut milk 1 cup	1	5	0	77
5 a day salad (choose any 5 below)	6	15	5	70	Almond milk 1 cup	2	1	1	40
Spinach: 1 small bowl									
Pak choi: 3 heaped tbsp (shredded)					**Fruit**				
Lettuce (mixed): 1 small bowl					Apple	0	25	4	95
Swish chard: small bowl					Pear	1	27	6	101
Cucumber: 2-inch piece					Orange	1	15	3	62
Courgettes: half large					Raspberries 1/2 cup	1	7	4	32
Cabbage: 3 heaped tbsp (shredded)					Strawberries 1 cup	1	11	3	46
Broccoli: 2 spears					Avocado (medium)	3	12	10	232
Asparagus: 5 spears					Lemon	0	4	0	13
Celery: 3 sticks					Grapefruit (1/2 medium)	1	10	1	39
Pulses (cooked) 3 heaped tbsp*	3	8	4	45					
Kidney, broad, pinto, butter, borlotti,					**Snacks/other**				
black eye, lentils, chickpeas					Coconut yoghurt (125g)	4	1	1	229
					Mixed seeds (1/4 cup)	9	7	5	202
Oil/butter					10 half walnuts	3	3	1	132
Olive oil 1 tbsp	-	-	-	120	10 almonds	2	2	1	63
Coconut oil 1 tbsp	-	-	-	117	10 cashews	2	4	0	69
Avocado oil 1 tbsp	-	-	-	124	10 olives	0	1	1	40
Butter 1 tbsp	-	-	-	102	Flax seeds 1 tbsp	1	2	2	37
Flax seed oil 1 tbsp	-	-	-	114	Psyllium husk 1 tsp	-	4	4	8

* Pulses count as a maximum of 1 portion a day however much you eat as they don't give the same mix of nutrients as other veg.

Exercise and supplements

Exercise	Options	Mon	Tue	Wed	Thu	Fri	Sat	Sun
		Stretch / relaxation	H.I.I.T	Resistance	H.I.I.T	Resistance	Endurance	Rest
	1	Yoga / Tai Chi / meditation / stretch	20 mins Indoor / outdoor interval (sprints / walking / cycling / elliptical trainer / skipping)	Free weights / body weight exercises	20 mins Indoor / outdoor interval (sprints / walking / cycling / elliptical trainer / skipping)	Free weights / body weight exercises	up to 60 mins. jog	
	2	Walking / swimming	20 mins circuits / spinning / freestyle	BodyPump / circuits / power yoga	20 mins circuits / spinning / freestyle	BodyPump / circuits / power yoga	up to 60 mins. walk	

Drinks		Mon	Tue	Wed	Thu	Fri	Sat	Sun
	Ideas	2 X green tea	Lemon juice with h/w	Greens powder	Lemon juice with h/w	Greens powder	Lemon juice with h/w	2 X green tea
		1.5 litres of water	1.5 litres of water	1.5 litres of water	1.5 litres of water	1.5 litres of water	1.5 litres of water	1.5 litres of water

Supplements								
	Ideas	Multivitamin	Multivitamin	Multivitamin	Multivitamin	Multivitamin	Multivitamin	Multivitamin
		Probiotic	Probiotic	Probiotic	Probiotic	Probiotic	Probiotic	Probiotic
		Fish / flax seed oil	Fish / flax seed oil	Fish / flax seed oil	Fish / flax seed oil	Fish / flax seed oil	Fish / flax seed oil	Fish / flax seed oil

Detox								
	Ideas	Burdock root tea	Dandelion tea	Burdock root tea	Dandelion tea	Burdock root tea	Dandelion tea	Dandelion tea
		Psyllium husk	Flax seeds	Psyllium husk	Flax seeds	Psyllium husk	Flax seeds	Psyllium husk

De-stress								
	Ideas	Hobbies	Meditation / yoga	Hobbies	Meditation / yoga	Hobbies	Meditation / yoga	Hobbies
		Music	Reading	Cinema	Socialising	Music	Massage	Reading

Your Food Plan. Monitor carbs daily or two non-consecutive fat burn days. Maintain sufficient calorie, protein and fibre intake.

Food		Mon	Tue	Wed	Thu	Fri	Sat	Sun
Carbs	Grams							
Breakfast								
Options	1							
	2							
	3							
	4							
	5							
Lunch								
Options	1							
	2							
Dinner								
Options	1							
	2							
Snacks								
Options	1							
	2							
	3							
	4							
	5							

Portions if using your hand – Protein: size and thickness of palm. **Starchy carbs/fruit:** size of your fist. **Non starchy veg:** unlimited. **Cheese:** size of thumb

Red meat and oily fish – Red meat: no more than 70g per day. **Oily fish** (140g per portion): men up to 4 portions per week, women up to 2 portions per week.

89

Exercise and supplements

Exercise	Options		Stretch / relaxation	H.I.I.T	Resistance	H.I.I.T	Resistance	Endurance	Rest
			Mon	Tue	Wed	Thu	Fri	Sat	Sun
	1								
	2								

Drinks	Ideas		Mon	Tue	Wed	Thu	Fri	Sat	Sun

Supplements	Ideas	

Detox	Ideas	

De-stress	Ideas	

Chapter 15

Recipe ideas

Cooking some meals from scratch using mainly fresh ingredients is part of the process so you have a better idea and awareness of what you are eating. Somewhere along the line we have been convinced that we are too busy to even cook our own porridge, and yes, those sachets and pots are handy but some of them can be laden with added sugar. There are plenty of fast fresh food ideas online which you can dip in and out of. A few ideas to help kick-start the process are listed below.

Breakfast salad

Servings: 1
Prep: 3 mins
Ingredients:
- 1 large handful of mixed (red and green) lettuce leaves
- ½ small avocado, chopped
- ¼ red onion, chopped
- 1 teaspoon of apple cider vinegar
- 2 teaspoons of olive oil
- Salt and pepper to taste

Directions
Wash mixed lettuce leaves.
Mix vinegar, oil, salt and pepper together in a bowl, add lettuce and avocado and mix well – can be served with egg, smoked salmon, mackerel or sardines.

Honey salmon

Servings: 1
Prep: 5 mins **Cook:** 15–20 mins (depending on size of salmon)
Ingredients:
* ½ teaspoon of honey
* ½ teaspoon of soy or fish sauce
* Salmon fillet (or tofu)

Directions
Mix honey and soy sauce together. Spread sauce over salmon, oven bake or grill at medium heat. Serve with blanched pak choi or 5 a day salad.

Creamy mushrooms and veg

Servings: 1
Prep: 5 mins **Cook:** 5 mins **Ready in:** 10 mins
Ingredients:
* 1 teaspoon of oil
* 1 teaspoon of butter
* 1 cup of sliced mushrooms
* 2 tablespoons of whole milk
* ½ teaspoon of Dijon mustard
* 1 handful of chopped broccoli

Directions
Shallow boil broccoli. Cook mushrooms in oil until soft. Add butter and mustard, continue to stir. Add milk and stir well. Add salt and pepper to taste then serve mushrooms with broccoli.

Two superfoods on toast

Servings: 1
Prep: 1 min **Cook:** 4 mins (depending on how you like your eggs) **Ready in:** 5 mins
Ingredients:

- 1 slice of sourdough bread
- ¼ ripe avocado (2 tablespoons)
- 2 teaspoons of solid (but spreadable) organic coconut oil
- 2 eggs (can use cooked mackerel or sardines instead)

Directions
Hard boil eggs. Toast sourdough bread and allow to cool before spreading coconut oil on toast (tastes like butter, promise!). Mash and spread avocado on toast using fork. Cut eggs in half and place on top of avocado (cut side down).

Egg and veg

Servings: 1
Prep: 2 mins **Cook:** 4 mins (depending on how you like your eggs) **Ready in:** 6 mins
Ingredients:

- 2 eggs
- 1 tablespoon of oil
- ½ small onion chopped
- 1 Small handful of shredded spinach (or pak choi/swish chard)
- Pinch of chilli powder and salt to taste (optional)

Directions
Sauté onions in oil on medium heat in a frying pan. Reduce heat and add 2 (beaten) eggs. Add spinach just before eggs are cooked as desired.

Creamy green juice

Servings: 2
Prep: 5 mins **Ready in:** 15 mins
Ingredients:

- 1 kiwi
- 4–6 sticks of celery
- 1½–2 medium cucumbers
- ½ avocado, medium (ripe)
- 2 handfuls of spinach (or swiss chard)
- 1 teaspoon of super greens powder (optional)
- 1 apple or pear (optional)

Directions

Briefly soak all ingredients (except kiwi and avocado) in white vinegar (up to 10%) and water solution then rinse thoroughly. Juice cucumber, celery and spinach. Peel kiwi and avocado (remove stone). Place vegetable juice, kiwi and avocado into blender. Blend until smooth.

Juice can be stored in a dark airtight container, fill container to the brim and keep refrigerated. Ideally drink immediately or within 24 hours but can keep for up to 72 hours. You might notice a difference in taste the longer you wait to drink it. The moment you juice a fruit or vegetable, it starts to oxidise so some nutrients will be lost if not consumed straight away, but I would rather have a juice with less nutrients than no juice at all.

Home-made chilli seasoning
for meat, poultry or fish

Ingredients:
- 2 tablespoons of chilli powder
- 1 tablespoons of Himalayan salt
- 1 tablespoon of onion powder
- 1 tablespoon of celery powder
- 1 teaspoon of garlic powder
- 1 teaspoon of ginger powder

Directions
Combine ingredients, mix well and store in airtight container.

Vinaigrette salad dressing (for 5 a day salad)

Servings: 2–4
Ingredients:
- 1 teaspoon of dried mixed herbs
- 2 teaspoons of apple cider vinegar
- 1 teaspoon of Dijon mustard
- Juice of ½ a lemon
- 4 tablespoons of olive oil
- ½ a teaspoon of raw organic honey (optional)
- Salt and black pepper to taste

Directions
Squeeze lemon juice into cup. Add remaining ingredients and mix well. Keep refrigerated in glass bottle.

Raw vegetable wrap

Servings: 1
Prep: 5 mins **Ready in:** 7 mins
Ingredients:

- 1 large white cabbage leaf uncut (can use red cabbage)
- ¼ small red onion sliced
- 1 small carrot shredded
- 1 small handful of spinach
- 1 inch of cucumber, sliced
- 1 teaspoon of ground mixed seeds
- Pinch of dry mixed herbs
- 2 teaspoons of olive oil
- 1 teaspoon of apple cider vinegar
- ½ teaspoon of tamarind or soy sauce

Directions
Wash and prepare veg.

Mix dry herbs, ground seeds, olive oil, apple cider vinegar and tamarind or soy sauce together into a paste. Spread paste (or alternative pâté of choice) on the inside of cabbage leaf – leaf will have a natural curve. Place remaining vegetables inside cabbage leaf. Can be wrapped in foil and refrigerated.

Quick Thai red curry

Servings: 2
Prep: 15 **Cook:** 5 mins **Ready in:** 20 mins
Ingredients:

- ½ red bell pepper
- Juice of half a lime
- ½ small red onion, chopped
- ½ teaspoon of chilli powder
- 1 clove of garlic, chopped
- 1 chunk of fresh ginger (thumb size)
- 2 tablespoons of tomato puree
- Small handful of fresh coriander
- 1 tablespoon of fish or soy sauce
- 4 tablespoons of thick coconut milk
- ½ a stalk of fresh lemon grass (optional)
- 1 tablespoon of avocado (or olive) oil

Directions
Wash coriander leaves and prepare veg.

Blend all ingredients except oil into a paste (add water if too thick). Cook paste in oil for 2–3 minutes. Add choice of cooked prawns, meat or tempeh. Serve with 5 a day salad and/or basmati rice.

Sweet potato and bean soup

Servings: 2–4
Prep: 5 mins **Cook:** 25 mins **Ready in:** 30 mins (longer if using dry beans)
Ingredients:

* 1 tablespoon of oil
* 1 medium onion, finely chopped
* 1 sweet potato, peeled and diced
* 1 cup of stock (vegetable, chicken or beef stock)
* Black beans (or other beans), 400g can (drain and rinse)
* 1 fresh tomato
* Salt and pepper to taste

Directions
Blend tomato and set aside. Sauté onions in oil then add sweet potato and continue to stir. Add stock; bring to boil then simmer for 15 mins. Add beans and tomato.

Continue to simmer until sweet potato is soft. If using dry beans, use quick soak method and ensure beans are cooked through. Quick soak method – boil dry beans for 2 minutes in plenty of water. Let stand for 1 hour then rinse and cook beans until soft.

Fat burning vegetable soup

Servings: 4–6
Prep: 10 mins **Cook:** 15 mins **Ready in:** 25 mins
Ingredients:

- 1 tablespoon of oil
- 3 carrots, chopped
- 1 small onion, chopped
- 3 sticks of celery, chopped
- Shredded cabbage, 1 and a half cups
- 2 cups of stock (vegetable, chicken or beef stock)

Directions
Wash all vegetables.

In a large pot, sauté onions in oil for 2 minutes then add remaining vegetables and continue to stir. Add stock and simmer.

Once cooled, you can semi-blend soup using a hand blender. Soup can then be stored for a few days. Keep refrigerated.

Homemade pesto

Ready in: 15 mins

Ingredients:

- 2 handfuls of fresh basil leaves
- 1 small handful of fresh oregano leaves
- 1 handful of raw cashew nuts
- 1–2 cloves of garlic
- 6–10 tablespoons of olive oil
- ½ teaspoon of soy sauce (optional)
- Himalayan salt and black pepper to taste

Directions

Wash basil and oregano leaves.

Combine basil, oregano, cashew nuts and garlic into a food processor (or small blender) and process until mixture is coarse. Slowly add olive oil while you pulse the processor until mixture becomes a smooth paste. Remove from processor and stir in soy sauce then add salt and pepper to taste.

Store in glass bottle and keep refrigerated – can be used occasionally as a dip or spread.

References

1 http://www.menshealth.com/mhlists/muscle_building/Muscles_Need_More_than_Protein.php

2 Clissold, Lorraine. Why the Chinese don't count calories. 2008 ISBN 978-1-84529-842-5 P8

3 Clissold, Lorraine. Why the Chinese don't count calories. 2008 ISBN 978-1-84529-842-5 P8

4 http://www.nhs.uk/Conditions/vitamins-minerals/Pages/Vitamins-minerals.aspx

5 http://www.mayoclinic.org/healthy-living/weight-loss/in-depth/metabolism/art-20046508

6 Eades, Mary Dan. The Doctor's Complete Guide to Vitamins and Minerals 2000 ISBN: 9780440236450

7 Rose, Sara. Vitamins & Minerals: How to get the nutrients your body needs 2007 ISBN: 9780753716328

8 http://www.nhs.uk/Livewell/Goodfood/Pages/fish-shellfish.aspx

9 http://www.livestrong.com/article/499152-how-often-can-i-eat-liver-safely/

10http://webarchive.nationalarchives.gov.uk/+/www.dh.gov.uk/en/mediacentre/pressreleases/dh_124670

11 http://ndb.nal.usda.gov/ndb/

12 Recommended Daily Allowances (RDAs) for vitamins and minerals used instead of Dietary Reference Intakes (DRI) for ease of comparison

13 http://www.mayoclinic.org/healthy-living/nutrition-and-healthy-eating/in-depth/caffeine/art-20045678?pg=1

14 Source Information: "Higher antioxidant concentrations and less cadmium and pesticide residues in organically-grown crops: a systematic literature review and meta-analyses." Baranski, M. et al. British Journal of Nutrition, July 15th 2014

15 http://www.theguardian.com/environment/2014/jul/11/organic-food-more-antioxidants-study

16 Worthington et al. (From UK Soil Association Fact Sheet). Journal of Complimentary Medicine 7:2161- 2163 (2001)

17 http://articles.mercola.com/sites/articles/archive/2010/07/06/probiotics-bacteria-gut-digestive-health-immune-system.aspx

18 http://www.menshealth.co.uk/lose-weight/burn-fat/lose-more-weight-afterburn

19 blogs.abc.net.au/files/unswfatlossresearch.doc

20 http://newsroom.unsw.edu.au/news/how-burn-more-fat-less-effort

21 Research from the American Council on exercise

22 http://www.aworkoutroutine.com/how-much-muscle-can-you-gain/

23 Price, Weston A. June 2003. Nutrition and Physical Degeneration. Keats Pub; 6th edition

24 http://fitness.mercola.com/sites/fitness/archive/2012/11/09/high-intensity-training.aspx

25 http://ajcn.nutrition.org/content/87/3/778.full

26 http://www.ncbi.nlm.nih.gov/pubmed/3320694

27 http://diabetes.niddk.nih.gov/dm/pubs/insulinresistance/

28 http://www.bodybuilding.com/fun/issa7.htm

29 http://www.bodybuilding.com/teen/brent3.htm

30 http://www.obesityaction.org/educational-resources/resource-articles-2/general-articles/ghrelin-the-go-hormone

31 http://sleepfoundation.org/media-center/press-release/expert-panel-recommends-new-sleep-times

32 http://www.livestrong.com/article/402586-weight-lifting-for-better-sleep/

33 Glenville, Marilyn. Fat around the middle 2006 ISBN 978-1-85626-655-0 p. 11

34 Glenville, Marilyn. Fat around the middle 2006 ISBN 978-1-85626-655-0 p. 18 & 19

35 ^ Many Chemicals Accumulate in Our Fat Altern Med Rev Crinnion WJ.

36 Sears, Barry. Toxic Fat, when good fat turns bad. 2008 ISBN 978-1-4016-0429-5

37 http://www.rsc.org/chemistryworld/News/2009/August/27080901.asp

38 http://cen.acs.org/articles/87/i35/Cost-REACH-Underestimated.html

39 http://drhyman.com/blog/2012/02/20/how-toxins-make-you-fat-4-steps-to-get-rid-of-toxic-weight/

40 http://www.nhs.uk/chq/pages/1141.aspx?categoryid=51

41 http://www.hsph.harvard.edu/nutritionsource/carbohydrates/fiber/

42 http://www.nhs.uk/Conditions/Constipation/Pages/Introduction.aspx

43 Sears, Barry. Toxic Fat, when good fat turns bad. 2008 ISBN 978-1-4016-0429-5

44 http://www.nhs.uk/Livewell/5ADAY/Pages/Whatcounts.aspx

45 http://www.soilassociation.org/whatisorganic/organicfood/organicnutrition

46 http://www.alive.com/articles/view/22343/liver_kidney_cleansing

47 http://www.theguardian.com/lifeandstyle/2006/feb/11/healthandwellbeing.health

48 http://articles.mercola.com/sites/articles/archive/2012/01/12/aha-position-on-omega-6-fats.aspx

49 http://articles.mercola.com/sites/articles/archive/2015/02/02/anti-inflammatory-foods-herbs-spices.aspx

50 http://www.marksdailyapple.com/what-does-it-mean-to-be-fat-adapted/#axzz3KUZYN94F

51 http://www.diabetes.co.uk/body/insulin.html

52 http://diabetes.niddk.nih.gov/dm/pubs/insulinresistance/

53 Sears, Barry. Toxic Fat, when good fat turns bad. 2008 ISBN 978-1-4016-0429-5

54 http://healthyeating.sfgate.com/difference-between-sucrose-glucose-fructose-8704.html

55 Raben A, Vasilaras TH, Moller AC, Astrup A. Sucrose compared with artificial sweeteners: different effects on ad libitum food intake and body weight after 10 wk of supplementation in overweight subjects. Am J Clin Nutr 2002;76:721–9.

56 http://hyper.ahajournals.org/content/42/4/474.abstract?ijkey=eab2f1866bc1d4be5c059eede19c7d066da6df0d&keytype2=tf_ipsecsha

57 Masuo K, Kawaguchi H, Mikami H, Ogihara T, Tuck ML. Serum uric acid and plasma norepinephrine concentrations predict subsequent weight gain and blood pressure elevation. Hypertension 2003;42:474–80.

58 http://www.who.int/mediacentre/news/releases/2015/sugar-guideline/en/

59 http://www.dailymail.co.uk/health/article-2113073/Healthy-bars-Some-sugar-Kit-Kat.html

60 http://www.dailymail.co.uk/news/article-2421381/Shocking-foods-contain-far-sugar-Krispy-Kreme-doughnut.html

61 http://www.dailymail.co.uk/health/article-2301135/15-WORST-health-drinks-Orange-juice-Innocent-smoothies-sugar-13-Hobnobs-3-half-doughnuts.html

62 http://www.which.co.uk/documents/pdf/cereal-bars-full-report-293495.pdf

63 http://www.mcdonalds.co.uk/ukhome/more-food/desserts-treats.html

64 http://www.greenandblacks.co.uk/our-range/product-information

65 http://www.innocentdrinks.co.uk/things-we-make/our-smoothies/super-smoothie/antioxidant

66 https://www.fatsecret.com/calories-nutrition/generic/cake-cupcake-with-icing

67 http://www.quakeroats.com/products/hot-cereals/instant-oatmeal-cups/apples-and-cinnamon.aspx

68 http://www.yoplait.com/products/yoplait-light

69 http://www.dailymail.co.uk/health/article-2033234/Shocking-levels-salt-fat-favourite-takeaway.html

70 http://www.telegraph.co.uk/news/health/news/10677838/Sugar-levels-in-popular-food-and-drink-products.html

71 http://www.sugarstacks.com/sauces.htm

72 http://www.telegraph.co.uk/news/health/10716212/How-much-sugar-is-in-your-healthy-brown-and-wholemeal-bread.html

73 http://energydrink-uk.redbull.com/red-bull-calories

74 http://www.coca-cola.co.uk/drinks/coca-cola/coca-cola/#TCCC

75 http://www.dentalhealth.org/uploads/download/resourcefiles/download_19_1_Sugar-Table.pdf

76 http://www.euronews.com/2015/03/06/the-who-suggests-we-eat-50g-of-sugar-per-day-but-how-much-is-that-exactly/

77 http://www.nhs.uk/Livewell/loseweight/Pages/Appleorpear.aspx

78 http://diabetes.niddk.nih.gov/dm/pubs/insulinresistance/

79 http://www.theguardian.com/society/2013/mar/20/sugar-deadly-obesity-epidemic

80 http://fitness.mercola.com/sites/fitness/archive/2013/05/17/intermittent-fasting-diet.aspx

81 http://www.huffingtonpost.com/riva-greenberg/gl-and-gi_b_863126.html

82 http://www.dummies.com/how-to/content/the-gl-diet-for-dummies-cheat-sheet.html

83 http://www.health.harvard.edu/newsweek/Glycemic_index_and_glycemic_load_for_100_foods.htm

84 http://lpi.oregonstate.edu/infocenter/foods/grains/gigl.html

85 http://authoritynutrition.com/how-many-carbs-per-day-to-lose-weight/

86 http://www.nhs.uk/change4life/Pages/five-a-day-portion-sizes.aspx

87 http://www.diabetes.co.uk/insulin/insulin-sensitivity.html

88 http://www.mayoclinic.org/healthy-living/nutrition-and-healthy-eating/in-depth/high-fiber-foods/art-20050948

89 Lebovka, Nikolai (Editor), Vorobiev, Eugene (Editor), Chemat, Farid (Editor). Enhancing Extraction Processes in the Food Industry (Contemporary Food Engineering) (2011) p. 478. ISBN 978-1-4398-4593-6.

90 http://www.theguardian.com/environment/2010/jan/23/margarine-butter-health-wars

91 http://www.livestrong.com/article/557726-eat-fat-to-burn-fat/

92 http://www.mensfitness.com/nutrition/what-to-eat/eat-fat-to-slim-down

93 http://www.shape.com/weight-loss/food-weight-loss/ask-diet-doctor-latest-science-belly-fat

94 http://www.wakehealth.edu/News-Releases/2006/Trans_Fat_Leads_To_Weight_Gain_Even_on_Same_Total_Calories,_Animal_Study_Shows.htm

95 http://www.ncbi.nlm.nih.gov/pubmed/16531187

96 http://www.nhs.uk/conditions/metabolic-syndrome/Pages/Introduction.aspx

97 http://www.mayoclinic.org/healthy-living/weight-loss/in-depth/weight-loss/art-20047342

98 Pool, Robert (2001). Fat: fighting the obesity epidemic. Oxford [Oxfordshire]: Oxford University Press. p. 68. ISBN 0-19-511853-7.

99 http://www.mayoclinic.org/medical-professionals/clinical-updates/endocrinology/what-new-adipose-tissue

100 http://www.cosmopolitan.com/health-fitness/news/a34423/how-often-to-weigh-yourself/

101 http://www.livestrong.com/article/296653-how-many-calories-does-drinking-one-glass-of-water-burn/

102 http://www.nhs.uk/Livewell/Goodfood/Pages/eggs-nutrition.aspx

103 https://www.bhf.org.uk/news-from-the-bhf/news-archive/2015/may/eggs-and-cholesterol

104 http://www.diabetes.co.uk/natural-therapies/cinnamon.html

105 http://articles.mercola.com/sites/articles/archive/2015/02/09/sprouts-nutrition.aspx

106 Smedman A, Vessby B. Conjugated linoleic acid supplementation in humans--metabolic effects. Lipids. 2001 Aug;36(8):773-81.

107 Nuria Laso, et al. Effects of milk supplementation with conjugated linoleic acid (isomers cis-9, trans-11 and trans-10, cis-12) on body composition and metabolic syndrome components. Br J Nutr. 2007 Oct;98(4):860-7.

108 http://www.womenshealthmag.com/weight-loss/probiotics

109 http://www.livestrong.com/article/495436-catechin-weight-loss/

110 http://ajcn.nutrition.org/content/82/1/41.abstract

111 http://ajcn.nutrition.org/content/87/1/23.short

112 http://jn.nutrition.org/content/134/3/586.short

113 http://ajcn.nutrition.org/content/82/1/41.full

114 http://www.theguardian.com/business/2010/nov/23/food-book-extract-felicity-lawrence

115 http://www.kelloggs.co.uk/en_GB/our-history.html

116 http://www.nhs.uk/Livewe

ll/alcohol/Pages/calories-in-alcohol.aspx

117 http://youngwomenshealth.org/2013/10/31/pms/

118 http://www.shape.com/lifestyle/mind-and-body/why-you-gain-weight-your-period

119 http://omronhealthcare.com/wp-content/uploads/hbf-514c-instruction-manual.pdf

120 http://omronhealthcare.com/wp-content/uploads/hbf-514c-instruction-manual.pdf

121 http://www.webmd.com/diet/calories-chart

* Registration, Evaluation, Authorisation & restriction of Chemicals (REACH) - A European Union regulation which addresses the production and use of chemical substances.

Last access date for website references 16th August 2015

www.ingramcontent.com/pod-product-compliance
Lightning Source LLC
Chambersburg PA
CBHW060417290526
45791CB00002B/792